Discovery and Healing

David Vaughn, MD

Discovery and Healing

Reflections on Five Decades of Hematology/
Oncology at the Perelman School of
Medicine at the University of Pennsylvania

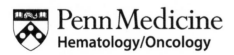 **Penn Medicine**
Hematology/Oncology

Penn Medicine Division of Hematology/Oncology
Philadelphia

Distributed by
University of Pennsylvania Press
Philadelphia, Pennsylvania 19104-4112
www.upenn.edu/pennpress

Printed in the United States of America on acid-free paper
10 9 8 7 6 5 4 3 2 1

ISBN 9780812225273 (Paperback)
ISBN 9780812298604 (Ebook)

For Annie, my astonishing wife

The noblest question in the world is:
What good may I do in it?

—BENJAMIN FRANKLIN

CONTENTS

FOREWORD

A few years ago, while many of us from the Hematology/Oncology Division were gathered in the Jordan Medical Education Center Atrium for a memorial service for Dr. Richard "Buz" Cooper, I realized with some urgency that a history of our remarkable division had to be written. Urgent because Buz, our very first division chief of Hematology/Oncology, had just died, and those who were gathering to remember and honor him were in the room where it happened—that is, they were there when it all began. That evening, Jim Hoxie, Dupont Guerry, Joel Bennett, Skip Brass, John Glick, and so many others shared stories about the history and the beginning days of our glorious division. Hearing them speak so eloquently, I committed myself to making sure we captured in writing their stories and our remarkable fifty-year history. What I did not know was that Dr. David Vaughn, an internationally recognized expert in testicular cancer and a twenty-five-year faculty member in the division, would ultimately take on this important project and use his precious sabbatical time to write our history.

The Hematology/Oncology Division began in 1971–1972, the same year the National Cancer Act was enacted. It is remarkable to reflect on the major advances in our understanding of cancer over the past fifty years and the translation of this research into new treatments that improve the lives of patients with cancer. This division—the physicians, scientists, researchers, nurses, and staff—has played a leading role in these advances. At the same time, the division has contributed so much to advancing our understanding of hemostasis, coagulation, and HIV. Education and training are also a vital part of the division, and it is remarkable to reflect on how many future leaders across the country were trained here.

Today, the Hematology/Oncology Division employs more than 650 staff, faculty, nurses, and clinicians; supports more than 200,000 annual outpatient visits; and has over 100 open clinical trials. The division is nationally and internationally renowned for cutting-edge translational research such as CAR-T cells and for providing exceptional and compassionate clinical care. The deep expertise of the faculty has positioned the division, along with the Abramson Cancer Center, to develop and test new cancer therapies that have led to numerous FDA-approved drugs and new approaches to diagnosing and treating benign hematological conditions. To date, all the outstanding directors of the Abramson Cancer Center have been faculty members in the Hematology/Oncology Division.

We celebrate the Fiftieth Anniversary of the Hematology/Oncology Division with this book, lovingly written by our own David Vaughn. In this beautifully written book, David combines his own journey as a medical oncologist in the Hematology/

Oncology Division with a look back at how we started and where we are today.

In the history of this division, we have had four division chiefs—Dr. Richard "Buz" Cooper, Dr. Sanford "Sandy" Shattil, Dr. Stephen Emerson, and me, appointed in 2007. It has been a privilege and honor to serve as a division chief of this most remarkable and special division. The members of the division have and are making a difference every day, and I could not be prouder of all that we have achieved together during this transformational time for our field. I hope you enjoy this book as much as I did.

With gratitude and appreciation,
Lynn Schuchter, MD
C. Willard Robinson Professor of Medicine
Chief, Hematology/Oncology Division
The Perelman School of Medicine at the University of
Pennsylvania
and the Abramson Cancer Center

PREFACE

"We have to move to Philadelphia!" It was the autumn of 1989 and my wife, Annie, then a third-year pediatric resident at Mt. Sinai Hospital in New York City, had just returned from spending the day at Children's Hospital of Philadelphia (CHOP) interviewing for a fellowship position in pediatric hematology/oncology. She was giddy with excitement, having met with some of the giants in the field. "I loved it! Everyone was so great. And they offered me a position!"

At the time, I was a third-year internal medicine resident at the New York Hospital–Cornell Medical Center. When I started my internship in July 1987, my first attending was Roy Silverstein, a rising star in the field of hematology. He was the kind of physician that I wanted to become. His teaching rounds were always interesting and informative, even for an exhausted intern. In addition, Roy was a brilliant scientist whose laboratory was making important discoveries about the biology of platelets and endothelium in the development of atherosclerosis. During the third year of residency we had a three-month "research block," and I asked Roy if I could spend it in his laboratory. It is hard to accomplish much in the lab in such a short time, especially with no prior bench training, but I did my best to study a protein called lysosome-associated membrane protein-2, or LAMP-2, on the surface of platelets. I can't say I was a natural, but Roy was always patient and encouraging. When I told him that I wanted to be a hematologist and that Annie wanted to be at CHOP, he told me I should train at the University of Pennsylvania.

I vividly remember my interview day at Penn. I met with several of the hematologists and felt like the day was going well. Then I met with the hematologist Doug Cines. I was feeling perhaps a bit too relaxed, and when Cines asked me what I saw myself doing in five years, I gave him my well-practiced answer: "I plan a career in academic hematology where I spend half my time in laboratory research and half my time in clinical medicine, and do a lot of teaching on the side." He looked at me quizzically. "Not possible," he replied. "You need to choose. Are you going to be a lab scientist or a clinician? You can't do both." I left the interview feeling foolish and was sure that I had blown my chance. But a few weeks later I was called by Sanford Shattil, Chief of Penn's Division of Hematology/Oncology, who offered me a position in their fellowship program. I was thrilled and accepted it on the spot, while Annie could not have been more pleased. We were moving to Philly.

Fast-forward more than thirty years, and we are still here. I am a medical oncologist, not a hematologist. I am a clinician-educator, not a laboratory scientist. I have been fortunate to be a member of a most remarkable Division of Hematology/Oncology. It is a Division that places great value on superb clinical care. Our faculty have made some of the most important scientific and clinical discoveries in the fields of hematology and medical oncology. We have a world-class fellowship program that attracts the best and the brightest graduating internal medicine residents and a faculty dedicated to their training.

One of the aspects of my career that I enjoy most is working side by side with our first-year fellows in my genitourinary oncology clinic. I take the responsibility of mentorship very seriously, and I have high expectations of the fellows. I model this experience after my own clinical apprenticeship working with John Glick during my second and third years of fellowship. Back in the day, Glick would invite one of the second- or third-year fellows to partner with him in clinic. It was a demanding but transformational experience. I learned how to care for patients with cancer in Glick's clinic. He was (and is) a phenomenal clinician. He also made seminal contributions to the field of breast cancer and lymphoma, served as Director of Penn's Comprehensive Cancer Center for twenty-one years, was President of the American Society of Clinical Oncology in 1996, and had the vision for the state-of-the-art ambulatory cancer center where we now practice. His portrait on the first floor of this building is a testament to his unparalleled contributions.

One day in clinic with one of the first-year fellows, we were evaluating a patient with enlarged lymph nodes. As I reviewed the case with the fellow, I made a teaching point about palpating lymph nodes and differentiating a benign node from a malignant one. "Let me teach you something that John Glick taught me when I was a fellow training in his clinic years ago." And the fellow responded, "Who's John Glick?" I then realized that institutional memory is indeed short.

Soon thereafter I was meeting with our Division Chief, Lynn Schuchter. Alan Schreiber, one of the founding members of the

Division who had a remarkable career at Penn as a laboratory hematology researcher, had recently died. Lynn and I were discussing Alan's death and memorial service and the lovely tribute that our colleague Charles Abrams wrote about Alan and his life. Our first Division Chief, Richard "Buz" Cooper, had died the previous year. Lynn mentioned that these deaths got her thinking about how important it would be to have a written history of the Division. I have always enjoyed reading about the history of medicine and pride myself on having a solid liberal arts education. After thinking about this for a couple of days, I told Lynn that I was going to write the history. I had a three-month sabbatical planned from July through September 2018, and I decided to spend it working on this project. My goal would be to document for future generations the stories and contributions of the people who have made our Division so exceptional. But I would necessarily have to be selective. I could not include information about every faculty member and every scientific discovery over the past five decades. For example, we have an incredible group of junior faculty who are the future of the Division, many of whom are not mentioned in this book. Perhaps in ten years one of them will update this history to document their remarkable accomplishments.

When the Division was established in 1972, there were 5 faculty members. We now have more than 120 and counting, making us larger than many departments of medicine. Our faculty have contributed to many of the important advances in hematology and cancer medicine over the past five decades. Most recently, Division faculty were instrumental in developing and gaining Food and Drug Administration (FDA) approval for a revolutionary new form of cancer immunotherapy called chimeric antigen receptor T cell (CAR-T) therapy. CAR-T is an excellent example of what can be achieved in medicine when innovative and hard-working faculty and staff are committed to collaborative discovery and healing.

The Division has evolved from a small group of laboratory hematologists to a large, complex organization that provides comprehensive clinical care to patients with benign blood disorders, hematological malignancies, and solid tumors at both our main patient care and clinical research center at the Hospital of the University of Pennsylvania, as well at Pennsylvania Hospital, Penn Presbyterian Medical Center, and affiliated centers in Philadelphia and the surrounding suburbs. The Division has world-class fundamental laboratory and translational researchers making discoveries at the cutting edge of medicine. Our fellowship training program in Hematology/Oncology is the crown jewel of the Division. To understand how we arrived at this extraordinary time and place, it is helpful to start at the beginning.

ONE

Before the Division

In 2015, the Perelman School of Medicine at the University of Pennsylvania celebrated its 250th Anniversary. The fascinating and rich history of the nation's first school of medicine has been well documented in several volumes, most recently in the superb book *To Spread the Light of Knowledge: 250 Years of the Nation's First Medical School*.[1]

Contributions to the field of hematology by Penn physicians date back to the earliest days of the medical school. John Conrad Otto, a graduate of the Penn medical school in 1796, practiced medicine at Pennsylvania Hospital, the nation's first hospital. In 1803, he published "An Account of an Hemorrhagic Disposition in Certain Families" in the *Medical Repository*, the first American medical journal.[2] In this paper, he described a New Hampshire family whose men had a hemorrhagic bleeding disorder. Otto called these men "bleeders." Thus, he was the first to describe the hereditary basis of a bleeding disorder that would later be known as hemophilia.

From 1885 to 1889, the great William Osler was Professor of Clinical Medicine at the University of Pennsylvania. Osler has been called America's first hematologist (despite his Canadian roots). He brought the first microscope to the Hospital of the University of Pennsylvania (HUP) and was Penn's first hematologist, before hematology was even an established discipline. His contributions to hematology were many, including identifying platelets as a normal component of blood and relating their function to clot formation. I think Osler would be pleased that years later a major field of investigation in the Division is the understanding of the biology and function of platelets as they relate to human disease.

William Williams, a 1949 graduate of Penn's School of Medicine, formally established hematology as a discipline at Penn. He was Professor of Medicine and Chief of the Hematology Section until 1969 when he left to become Chair of the Department of Medicine at the State University of New York Upstate Medical Center and eventually Dean of its College of Medicine. His laboratory research focused on the biochemical basis of blood coagulation, and he was the first to show that Russell's viper venom initiated blood clotting.[3] However, he is perhaps best known as the founding editor of the textbook *Hematology*. When he was editor in chief of the fourth edition, the book was renamed *Williams Hematology* in honor of his decades of contributions. When I started my Hematology/Oncology fellowship at Penn, I purchased *Williams Hematology*, unaware that Williams spent much of his career at Penn. Indeed, institutional memory is short.

Frank Gardner, another famous hematologist, came to Penn in 1966 from Boston. Initially at the Thorndike Memorial Laboratory and Boston City Hospital, he later became a hematologist at the Peter Bent Brigham Hospital. Gardner was Professor of Medicine at the University of Pennsylvania School of Medicine and led hematology at Presbyterian Hospital from 1966 to 1975. Along with his fellow Scott Murphy, who years later was an adjunct faculty member of our Division, Gardner was the first to demonstrate that platelets stored for four to five days at room temperature lasted longer in the circulation than did platelets stored at 4 degrees centigrade.[4] In addition, Gardner had a controversial reputation for his clinical and teaching style.

Andrew Schafer, a well-known hematologist who graduated from Penn's School of Medicine in 1973, recalled for me a transformational experience when he was a fourth-year medical student on a hematology elective at Presbyterian Hospital and Gardner was his attending. "Frank Gardner was one of the giants of hematology. Frank was also a giant, physically. He was 6 feet 6 or 7 inches. He was very stout and was an incredibly imposing and intimidating figure. He'd always wear a bow tie and a sparkly white shirt. His white coat was always completely ironed, and he was very formal. My first assigned patient to consult on was a young guy with sickle cell disease who spent much of his life in the hospital because of recurrent infections. Afternoon rounds were held at the nursing station, standing up. There was no conference room. Literally, there was an entourage, several fellows and residents, and I was at the bottom of the pecking order. He required that we present the cases without notes, including lab data. I went through all of these and got through the presentation. He had this real booming voice, and he said, looking down at me, if you could imagine, 'Do you have any questions?' I didn't know what he meant. 'What do you mean questions?' 'Well, do you have any questions about this patient that you just worked up?' 'Dr. Gardner, I know that sickle cell patients are prone to infections. It just seems to me that this young man has spent half his life in the hospital with bacterial infections. I guess my question is why.' There was this long pause. Absolute silence and he was just glaring at me. Finally, he yelled out at the top of his lungs, 'Well, damn it, Schafer, find out!'"

Schafer recalled how that afternoon Gardner invited him to his office where they discussed the possible mechanisms that might be responsible for recurrent infections in patients with sickle cell disease, and later they studied the patient's neutrophils in his laboratory. Schafer credits his interactions with Gardner as transformative: "The idea, just the thought that I could actually observe a problem with a patient and be able to take that question to the bench, and to try to figure it out, was so incredibly powerful and seductive. At that moment, I decided that I was going to go into hematology, because it was relatively easy to study blood and very interesting. Secondly, I was going to do research. Very few people have an epiphany moment like that."[5]

———

Penn also has played an important role in cancer medicine over the years. For many years the treatment of cancer was under the auspices of surgeons since this was the only treatment available. Cancer surgery has a vivid history at Penn. In 1889, the great American painter Thomas Eakins painted *The Agnew Clinic* to honor Penn surgeon David Hayes Agnew. In the painting Agnew is performing a partial mastectomy on a woman with breast cancer. The painting highlights surgical advances in anesthesia and antisepsis, and stands in stark contrast to Eakins's earlier painting *The Gross Clinic*.

Penn also pioneered the use of radiation to treat cancer. Henry Pancoast, who in 1912 was appointed as the first Professor of Roentgenology in the United States, was an early practitioner of radiation to treat leukemia and lymphoma.[6] He also was among the first to describe the leukemogenic effects of radiation. Among many contributions, Pancoast described the lung tumor that bears his name, the Pancoast tumor, a classic form of lung cancer arising in the apex of the lung and often associated with Horner's syndrome.

Unlike surgery, medical oncology is a relatively young discipline. Chemical warfare research during World War II led to the recognition of the profound cytotoxic effects of mustard gas on the bone marrow and lymph system. This discovery in turn led to the hypothesis that cytotoxic chemotherapy could be used to treat cancer. During the 1950s and 1960s, chemotherapy was starting to be utilized for the treatment of cancer. However, there was no discipline of medical oncology. Hematologists started using chemotherapy to treat hematologic malignancies, such as leukemia and lymphoma. Internists and surgeons became interested in using chemotherapy for the treatment of solid tumors.

The American Society of Clinical Oncology was founded in 1964. In 1968, the first Section of Oncology within a Department of Medicine was established at the University of Minnesota, led by B. J. Kennedy. His pioneering work in defining and establishing the field of medical oncology led to the flourishing of this new discipline. Nevertheless, it was not until 1972 that the American Board of Internal Medicine recognized medical oncology as a subspecialty. The first board examination in medical oncology was administered in 1973.[7]

At Penn during the 1960s and early 1970s, Robert Ravdin, a general surgeon and the son of the famous Penn surgeon Isidor Ravdin, established Penn's Neoplastic Chemotherapy Service under the auspices of the Department of Surgery. The internist Sylvan Eisman joined Ravdin in this effort. Clyde Barker, former Chair of the Department of Surgery at Penn, recalled that "the two of them had a floor in the Ravdin Building where they had this clinic where they were following patients with breast cancer and treating them with Cytoxan (cyclophosphamide) and other chemotherapeutic agents."[8] In 1960, they reported on the evaluation of cyclophosphamide, then a new chemotherapy agent, in "the first 143 patients with disseminated cancer treated at the Hospital of the University of Pennsylvania."[9] The year before, Ravdin presented these findings at the fiftieth annual meeting of the American Association of Cancer Research in Atlantic City. Despite being a surgeon, Ravdin was an early believer in the potential of chemotherapy in the treatment of cancer. In 1963, the newspaper the *Morning Call* reported that in a lecture to the Lehigh County Medical Society, Ravdin "told how chemotherapy can be used successfully in combatting the pain and distress of advanced cancer. . . . A pioneer in this method of cancer care, Dr. Ravdin is an internationally known authority on it."[10] In 1972 Ravdin, at age forty-two, died unexpectedly while attending a social function at Philadelphia's Union League. While Eisman and later Irving Berkowitz continued to administer chemotherapy to patients in their private practices, the opportunity now existed for formalizing at Penn the fledgling discipline of medical oncology.

TWO

The Early Years

In 1968, Arnold "Bud" Relman, a nephrologist and renal physiologist, was recruited to Penn to be the Frank Wister Thomas Professor of Medicine and Chair of the Department of Medicine. During his tenure as Chair, Relman recruited several Division chiefs to build the academic rigor of the Department. John Glick recalled, "Bud was purposely changing Penn from private practice into full-time academic medicine."[1] Relman would later leave Penn to become Editor in Chief of the *New England Journal of Medicine*, a position that he held for fourteen years.

Richard "Buz" Cooper trained at the National Cancer Institute under Drs. Emil Frei and Emil Freireich, pioneers in the use of combination chemotherapy to treat childhood acute leukemia. He then completed a hematology fellowship at Boston City Hospital, trained at the Thorndike Lab with James Jandl, and then joined the hematology faculty at Harvard. Jandl was a well-regarded laboratory hematologist, an expert in red blood cell biology, and the author of a comprehensive textbook of hematology. In 1971, Relman recruited Cooper to be Chief of the Section of Hematology at Penn, a position vacated by William Williams's recent departure. With Robert Ravdin's unexpected death and the growing interest both locally and nationally in formalizing medical oncology as an academic discipline, Relman expanded Cooper's role to be Chief of a newly formed, combined Section of Hematology/Oncology in 1972. (At Penn, Sections were subsequently called Divisions. For clarity, I will henceforth use the term Division of Hematology/Oncology.) At some institutions, medical oncology was established as a separate entity from hematology. At Johns Hopkins University, medical oncology became its own department outside of the Department of Medicine. At Penn and many other institutions, hematology and medical oncology were combined into one Division of Hematology/Oncology within the Department of Medicine.

Cooper viewed laboratory investigation in hematology as the top priority of the Division. His research focused on the biochemistry of red blood cell membranes, and his work contributed to our understanding of hemolytic anemia and hereditary spherocytosis. He was the first to demonstrate that alterations in the lipid composition in the membrane of the red blood cell resulted in spherocytosis.[2] Not surprisingly, Cooper focused his early recruitment efforts on hematologists who were physician-scientists with a primary interest in the laboratory.

One of his first recruits was Sanford "Sandy" Shattil. Shattil first crossed paths with Cooper when he was an internal medicine resident on the Harvard Medical Service at Boston City Hospital. Shattil recalled, "I thought that a career in cardiology was in my future, until a chance conversation with an attending physician, Dr. Richard 'Buz' Cooper, Chief of Hematology at the Thorndike

Memorial Laboratory. He invited me to consider a fellowship in hematology, a subject about which I knew little."[3] Shattil accepted the offer and trained in hematology at the Thorndike with Cooper as his mentor. Shattil then served with the Public Health Service in San Francisco. While there, Cooper invited Shattil to join the faculty of the newly formed Division at Penn, an offer he gladly accepted.

Shattil recalled for me his first impression of Philadelphia, a starkly different place from San Francisco. "Buz picked me up at the airport. The first thing I noticed was this incredible smoke over an area near the airport where they were compressing cars into small pieces of metal. I said, 'Is it like this here every day?' He said, 'Oh this is just a little fog. Don't worry about it.'" Although Shattil initially focused his research efforts on red blood cell membrane biology, the "fog" soon lifted, and his interests shifted to what was to become his lifelong research focus—platelets and their integrins in hemostasis, thrombosis, immunity, and inflammation.

Cooper also recruited Alan Schreiber who had trained in immunology with Michael Frank at the National Institutes of Health and later with the Harvard University rheumatologist Frank Austin.[4] Schreiber made seminal contributions to understanding antibody-mediated clearance of red blood cells and platelets by Fc receptors on macrophages. His work greatly enhanced our knowledge of immune thrombocytopenia and autoimmune hemolytic anemia. Schreiber spent his illustrious career at Penn. He died of Parkinson's disease in 2017 at age seventy-five.

James Wiley was an Australian hematologist who met Cooper while spending time at the Thorndike. He was living in London and planning to take a position there when he received a letter from Cooper offering him a position in the Division. He readily accepted and in 1972 joined the Division. Despite his junior status,

Cooper set him up with a laboratory and a technician. He collaborated with Cooper to characterize red blood cell membrane cation transport and lipid metabolism, contributing to our understanding of hereditary spherocytosis, hereditary stomatocytosis, and spur cell anemia.[5] Wiley was at Penn for four-and-a-half years before giving in to the pull of Australia. When I asked him why as an octogenarian he continued to work, he responded, "It keeps me young."[6]

Robert Colman, a Harvard-trained hematologist whose laboratory research focused on coagulation was another early member of the Division. He later moved to Temple University as Chief of Hematology. His textbook *Hemostasis and Thrombosis: Basic Principles and Clinical Practice* is considered a classic.

Peter Cassileth, a Columbia University–trained hematologist with an expertise in acute leukemia who was already at Penn when Cooper arrived, was tasked with coordinating the clinical programs of the Division. As a clinical researcher, Cassileth helped to define many of the principles in the treatment of acute myelogenous leukemia that are still in use today. He also established Penn's bone marrow transplantation program. In 1992, Cassileth left Penn to become Chief of Hematology/Oncology at the Sylvester Comprehensive Cancer Center at the University of Miami. In 2011, he died after a long battle with myelodysplastic syndrome and leukemia. In his honor, the University of Miami established the Peter A. Cassileth Award, given each year to a graduating fellow of the Hematology/Oncology Division who "demonstrates outstanding clinical judgment, enthusiasm for learning, and compassionate care."

Manfred Goldwein, a hematologist in private practice, was an adjunct member of the Division who interacted extensively with faculty and fellows. Jane Alavi, the first woman in the Division, recalled that when she was a fellow, Goldwein taught her how to do sternal bone marrow aspirations of which he was a master.[7] Wiley recalled Goldwein as a consummate clinical hematologist. "At Hematology conference, we'd discuss a particular patient and review some of the landmark studies in the particular disease. When it came to management of the patient, everyone would have an opinion, and then finally we'd turn to Fred Goldwein and say, 'Well, now, what does the wise old man say?' He was the venerable . . . physician who had the last word on what you would actually do to manage the patient." When I was a first-year fellow in 1990, Goldwein was actively seeing patients and teaching fellows. In 1999, Goldwein died at age seventy-five.

As I learned more about Cooper, it became clear that he was a dynamic, energetic, and highly intelligent leader. Shattil told me, "Buz Cooper is the model of a mentor and division chief. He had an incredible ability to lead. He had a tremendous breadth of expertise. He did excellent basic science, and had a sharp clinical acumen, again primarily in hematology because that's what we all had been trained in at Boston City Hospital. He was a mentor par excellence. He supported us. He allowed us to do research, some in his lab, but he then allowed us to go out on our own. He was just a tremendous model for mentor. He was also a close friend to most of us."

Wiley remembered his years at Penn fondly and credits Cooper for giving him an opportunity in the Division. "I have run hematology departments in Australia at two different hospitals. I've always thought the best way to do things is how Buz brilliantly organized it. Buz is the most tremendous mentor and colleague, and he had a terrific enthusiasm to get things done. No problem was too great. He interacted very well with people. There was a terrific sense of purpose in the Division. It was really an amazing time."

Lawrence "Skip" Brass, who was a Hematology/Oncology fellow under Cooper and later joined the Division as an Assistant Professor of Medicine, recalled that faculty meetings in those early days were held at Cooper's house. "We would all have dinner at Buz's house and everybody could fit in the house easily. Can you imagine that happening now? Buz was a very charismatic person, and in no small part responsible for the fact that I chose to come here instead of going off to Harvard."[8]

James Hoxie, another Hematology/Oncology fellow who became an Assistant Professor of Medicine in 1982 under Cooper, recalled conferences that were run by Cooper. "There was a so-called weekly 'Breakfast with Buz' that we all loved. The fellows would present all the patients to Buz, and he would discuss each one. There was also a hematology conference every Friday where everybody went, and the fellows presented cases." He remembers that this conference caused "a lot of anxiety because you were grilled. . . . Buz came from Boston . . . a rigorous place. Fellows were supposed to sweat . . . but we sort of expected it and you always learned."[9] Wiley added, "Buz couldn't tolerate fools and there were a few occasions where he gave short shrift to visiting speakers who were not up to par."

Cooper remained Chief of the Division until 1985, when he left Penn to become Dean of the Medical School at the Medical College of Wisconsin. While at Wisconsin, after his tenure as Dean, he established and directed the Health Policy Institute for eleven years. Interestingly, he returned to Penn in 2005 as a Professor of Medicine and Senior Fellow in the Leonard Davis Institute of Health Economics where "he reinvented himself as one of the country's most controversial health services researchers."[10] In January 2016, Cooper died of pancreatic cancer at age seventy-nine. Soon after his death, his final work, *Poverty and the Myths of*

Health Care Reform, was published. In this book, Cooper argued that our country's enormous health care spending is in large part related to poverty since the poor utilize disproportionately more health care resources, which drives up costs. Michael M. E. Johns, President and CEO of Emory Healthcare, wrote that Cooper's book was "an extremely important, brilliantly told story that, if understood by more people, would bring major changes to our health care system by improving medical care and reducing costs."[11]

On September 23, 2016, Cooper's colleagues held a symposium in his honor on the Penn campus. The opening event was an Alumni Hematology Conference, with case presentations and, true

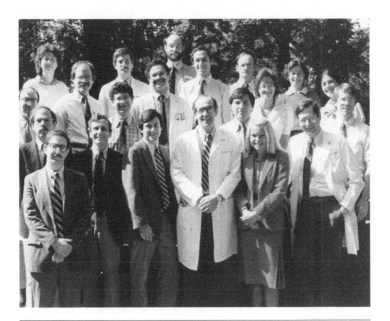

Figure 1. Division, 1982. Division Chief Richard "Buz" Cooper is in the front row, fourth from left.

to Cooper's spirit, a vigorous discussion. This is the same Friday-afternoon conference format that Cooper initiated and made famous when he came to Penn in 1971. It was followed by a Policy Symposium entitled "Healthcare Workforce Policy: Balancing Quality, Costs, and the Impact of Poverty." The discussants were health policy experts and colleagues of Cooper. Following the symposium, there was a personal tribute to Cooper, with speakers including Shattil, Glick, and Hoxie. In his tribute, Hoxie discussed the impact Cooper had on him personally. He recalled, "In my first years at Penn and in my transition to the faculty there was no one more influential in giving me gentle and, at times when I needed it, firm guidance."

THREE

The First Oncologist

Buz Cooper recognized the importance of medical oncology and the lack of real expertise in the Division. He knew that as a hematologist he needed a formally trained medical oncologist to partner with him and develop the medical oncology side of the Division. He found such a partner in John Glick.

Glick was the son of a prominent Manhattan dermatologist. He graduated from Columbia's College of Physicians and Surgeons where he remained for his internal medicine residency. However, while he was a resident, the Vietnam War was in full force. At the time, to avoid going to Vietnam, candidates from the top medicine residency programs applied to the National Institutes of Health (NIH) for fellowship training. Glick was accepted into the training and research program at the National Cancer Institute (NCI). "I was a clinical associate first on the Leukemia Service and then in the Medicine Branch. My attendings were [Vincent] DeVita, [Paul] Carbone, [Philip] Shein, [Robert] Young,

[Bruce] Chabner, [Brigid] Leventhal, and [George] Canellos."[1] These were the giants in the newly established, evolving field of medical oncology. At the NCI from 1971 to 1973, Glick became a medical oncologist who recognized the importance of well-designed, carefully performed cancer clinical trials.

In his book *Stay of Execution: A Sort of Memoir*, the political analyst and newspaper columnist Stewart Alsop who was battling leukemia at the NCI in the early 1970s described his oncologist. "Dr. Glick seemed surprisingly young.... He was very thin, with side burns, a white coat, a tie and a blue button-down shirt, and a quick and easy manner. It was very soon clear that he was very intelligent, highly competent, and—this can be even more important to a patient whose life is at risk—a nice man and a good man."[2]

In 1973, Glick left the NCI and went to Stanford University for another year of fellowship training under Henry Kaplan and Saul Rosenberg, two pioneers in the treatment of Hodgkin's disease. While at Stanford, Glick's career goals began to crystallize. "I wanted to be in academic medicine with a combination of seeing patients and doing clinical research, which was a job description that did not exist at the time." He continued, "DeVita started giving my name out, and I got calls from across the country: Columbia, University of Chicago, Stanford." He was close to signing on with the University of Chicago when he received a call from Cooper. 'I've heard from Vince [DeVita]. My name's Buz Cooper. I'm head of Hematology/Oncology at Penn. We don't have any oncologists.'"

The two met for the first time soon thereafter in Chicago at the meeting of the American Society of Hematology. Glick recalled the meeting: "Buz had no oncologists at Penn. He needed an oncologist. I went to the coffee shop at the Marriott. I sit at a table for two, and this guy comes in. He was tall, gaunt, with a scraggly goatee. He sat down at a table with those piercing eyes. He asked me about myself, he asked me what I wanted to do, and I described my vision of clinical research and taking exquisite care of patients. Maybe a week or two later, he calls and says, 'John, will you come out for a visit? I'll pay your way.' I said, 'Sure, but I'm very close to making a decision at another institution.' He said, 'Just come out and chat with me.'"

Glick remembered his first visit to Penn and, in particular, the spirited atmosphere. "I came out and stayed at Buz's house in Swarthmore. The next day I interviewed with Peter [Cassileth], Sandy [Shattil], [Alan] Schreiber, Buz, Jim Wiley. They took me to Al's for lunch. Everybody in the division went to Al's for lunch, which was a greasy spoon on Walnut Street. And then I went to Hematology conference. I thought I had entered a lunatic asylum. DuPont [Guerry, who at the time was a fellow] was presenting; he was three words into his presentation and he was interrupted. Schreiber and Sandy were going at each other. Buz is hardly listening to the presentation, saying, 'This is the worst peripheral smear I have ever seen in my life. Who made this peripheral smear?' DuPont is as calm as can be. Peter is trying to get a word in. I don't remember the case. Unbelievable. But there was an air of excitement. Penn was recruiting very talented young people under the leadership of the Chairman of Medicine, Arnold 'Bud' Relman. It was an all-star cast that was being recruited. There was an energy about this place."

Soon after this visit, Glick received a late-night phone call from Cooper. "Buz says, 'I'm offering you a job. I want you to see patients and I want you to do clinical research.' I said, 'That's great. Buz, can we talk about salary?' He said, 'Salary? What salary? Okay. I'll offer you $23,000.' Finally, we settled on $26,000, plus he paid me one month early to cover the cost of my move."

When he joined the Division in 1974, Glick was the only bona fide medical oncologist at Penn. He has been at Penn ever since.

Glick recalled his initial days at Penn. "Coming in the first day, Buz is on sabbatical and is nowhere to be found. Peter Cassileth is the acting chief. I walked into his office and said, 'Peter, where's my office?' He says, 'I don't have an office for you.' So I moved a desk into one of the clinic exam rooms. The first three days, the nurse and I washed the clinic. It was filthy. We couldn't get housekeeping to do it. We literally scrubbed the entire clinic."

As the only medical oncologist at Penn, Glick became very busy very fast. He established the first inpatient oncology unit, a four-bed unit on Dulles 3. "For four years I did virtually every oncology consult in the hospital. I treated brain tumors, I treated everything. I personally administered chemotherapy. I had neutropenic admissions. I had deaths from chemotherapy. I was in clinic four or five days a week. I never got home before 10 o'clock at night." At a tumor board conference, he proposed treating a young man with metastatic testicular cancer with a new chemotherapy agent, cisplatin, and was "laughed out of the room." Never one to be dissuaded, Glick treated and cured this patient.

Breast cancer was a major clinical interest, and Glick was at the forefront of this field and was in demand clinically. "My first day here I get a call from Bud Relman whose neighbor just had a radical mastectomy for breast cancer. 'Can I introduce you to her and will you take care of her?' She had twelve positive nodes. She was the first person in Philadelphia to get adjuvant chemotherapy for breast cancer. I gave her Alkeran for two years and chest wall and nodal radiation. She never recurred from her breast cancer but thirty-five years later died of a radiation-induced mesothelioma." When Gianni Bonadonna reported his trial of adjuvant cyclophosphamide, methotrexate, and 5-fluorouracil in women with node-positive breast cancer in 1976,[3] Glick became an early advocate for incorporation of adjuvant chemotherapy in the management of patients with breast cancer. He even started treating patients with node-negative breast cancer in 1982, years before the definitive randomized trials were published. Additionally, Glick and Robert Goodman, who was recruited to Penn in 1977 to become the first Chair of the Department of Radiation Oncology, were pioneers in the use of lumpectomy and radiation therapy for breast conservation, offering this approach to patients in Philadelphia as early as 1977, nearly a decade before the treatment was adopted in broader use. Glick also pioneered the integration of chemotherapy into breast conservation treatment.

Having trained with the world's experts in Hodgkin's disease at Stanford, Glick also focused on treating patients with lymphoma. He was the "go-to" oncologist in Philadelphia for patients with Hodgkin's disease and non-Hodgkin's lymphoma. "I started giving CHOP (a chemotherapy regimen of cyclophosphamide, doxorubicin, vincristine, and prednisone) in the late 1970s. Patients had these incredible responses." He led clinical trials in lymphoma through the Eastern Cooperative Oncology Group (ECOG), including the trial that established the standard (at the time) chemotherapy regimen for Hodgkin's disease.[4]

Glick also understood that many types of cancer were not curable with the drugs available at the time. Unlike common practice then, Glick believed in being honest and fully disclosing to a patient and family the diagnosis and prognosis. "I remember a patient with relapsed follicular lymphoma. I said, 'You're going to live for years but I can't cure your disease.' I was telling people the diagnosis and I was getting into trouble. The family said, 'You'll kill my mother if you tell her the diagnosis.'" Despite these pressures, he never withheld information from patients and families.

As he was breaking new ground in medical oncology at Penn, Glick stated that "Buz was supporting me in everything I did."

———

In 1971, President Richard Nixon signed into law the National Cancer Act. An important component of that act was funding to establish fifteen cancer centers across the country. In October 1971, Dean Alfred Gelhorn invited faculty from the School of Medicine to discuss the feasibility of creating a cancer center at the University of Pennsylvania. This initial meeting resulted in the submission of a Cancer Center Planning Grant which was successfully funded and set the stage for submission of the first Cancer Center Support Grant (CCSG), also known as the "core grant."[5]

Glick recalled that Cooper wrote the first core grant in 1973 and then subsequently planned and orchestrated the site visit. At a site visit, expert grant reviewers visit the institution to determine, among other things, if the submitting institution has the resources and wherewithal to accomplish what it proposes in the grant. Glick, who had agreed to come to Penn but had not yet started, remembers visiting Cooper the night before the first site visit. "I get to his house; it's the night before the site visit. He hands me the core grant; I have never seen it before. I said, 'Buz, this whole section of clinical research is impossible. You are proposing large-scale, randomized clinical trials in a single institution. You can't do it. What we should be doing are small trials to try and prove a point.' He said, 'Okay, John, you're presenting tomorrow.' He put me on the site visit agenda, no rehearsal, no slides. At the site visit, Buz said 'John, tell us about your concept for clinical research.'" At a blackboard, Glick outlined for the reviewers his vision for cancer clinical research at Penn. The core grant site visitors gave Glick his first NIH funding, which he held continuously for thirty-two years.

Penn's first CCSG was successfully funded in 1973, and Penn has had continuous grant funding through the CCSG mechanism ever since. The first of these grants was 155 pages and requested $3,190,823 for three years of funding. In contrast, Penn's 2020 CCSG application had 2,182 pages and requested $46,176,395 over five years.[6] In 1974, the University of Pennsylvania Cancer Center (UPCC) received "comprehensive" status, the highest given by the NCI. Peter Nowell, the Chair of the Department of Pathology who first described the Philadelphia chromosome in chronic myelogenous leukemia,[7] was named first Director of the UPCC. Cooper was his Associate Director. In 1975, Nowell stepped down as Director. Cooper, who was instrumental in securing funding of the first core grant and had demonstrated remarkable leadership as Division Chief, was named the next Director, a position he held until he left Penn in 1985. Cooper appointed Glick as his Associate Director for Clinical Research, a position that allowed Glick to develop his own administrative and leadership skills.

FOUR

The Division Grows

Under Buz Cooper's leadership, the Division began to grow, and fundamental hematology research was a priority. Cooper identified great potential in several of his Hematology/Oncology fellows and hired them to be part of his faculty. All would go on to distinguished careers as physician-scientists. In 1975, Joel Bennett completed his Hematology/Oncology fellowship at Penn and joined the faculty. As a fellow, he worked in Sandy Shattil's laboratory and developed his interest in platelet biology. Bennett recalled his early years as a junior faculty member in the Division. "It was a very fortunate time because nobody knew anything. It was easy to discover things. It was basic biochemistry. When I started to work in the lab, Sandy was my mentor. For a long time, we shared a lab, we shared technicians." Standing at a laboratory sink one day, Bennett had an idea. "I ran back to Buz's office and said, 'I got this project I want to do.' I told him what it was, and he said, 'Fine. Go do it.' It was amazing. I don't know where the idea came from."[1]

To understand the importance of Bennett's discovery, some background is helpful. In 1918, a Swiss pediatrician, Edward Glanzmann, described a group of patients who presented with bleeding and bruising of the mucous membranes and skin. These patients had normal platelet counts but clearly abnormal platelet function. This disorder became known as Glanzmann's thrombasthenia.[2] By the mid-1970s, investigators had demonstrated that these patients were deficient in two distinct, paired glycoproteins normally present on the surface of platelets and together designated glycoprotein (GP) IIb/IIIa (now known as integrin $\alpha IIb\beta_3$). However, the function of GP IIb/IIIa was not well understood. In 1979, Bennett demonstrated that fibrinogen binding to platelets required platelet activation and that platelet aggregation required fibrinogen binding.[3] He demonstrated that platelets from patients with Glanzmann's thrombasthenia had a hereditary deficiency and/or defect in GPIIb/IIIa, the fibrinogen receptor on the surface of the platelet. Bennett and colleague James Hoxie developed a monoclonal antibody to GP IIb/IIIa and demonstrated that this antibody blocked the binding of fibrinogen to this receptor.[4]

Thus, early in his career, Bennett made a major discovery that was central to understanding how platelets function and to understanding the pathophysiology of a previously unexplained disease, Glanzmann's thrombasthenia. Bennett's discovery laid the foundation for the eventual development of the first rationally designed antiplatelet agents to prevent and treat cardiovascular disease ($\alpha IIb\beta_3$ antagonists). In recognition of this seminal contribution, Bennett was awarded in 2010 (as the corecipient with Barry Coller) the prestigious Ernest Beutler Lecture and Prize by the American Society of Hematology. On September 7, 2017, the Penn-CHOP [Children's Hospital of Philadelphia] Blood Center held a symposium on thrombosis in celebration of Bennett's seventy-fifth birthday. Thrombosis experts from across the country, including Shattil and Coller, presented their research in honor of Bennett. Even into his late seventies, Bennett ran an NIH-funded laboratory, continued to make important discoveries related to platelet biology and function, and practiced benign hematology.

James Hoxie was drawn to hematology after a close cousin died of leukemia when he was a child. A graduate of Penn's medical school in 1976, Hoxie subsequently returned to Penn for a Hematology/Oncology fellowship and then joined the Division. Initially, his main interest was in the therapeutic use of monoclonal antibodies for leukemia. However, in the early 1980s, the development of a strange new disease changed his career focus. At that time, gay men presented with unusual infections, such as *Pneumocystis carinii* pneumonia. They also developed atypical malignancies, such as Kaposi's sarcoma, a disease previously seen only in the elderly. This unusual illness was originally called "gay-related immune deficiency," or GRID, but later became known as acquired immunodeficiency syndrome, or AIDS. In 1982, the first patient with AIDS was admitted to the Hospital of the University of Pennsylvania (HUP). At the time, Hoxie, while working in Buz Cooper's lab, was studying a white blood cell called a CD4 lymphocyte using a new experimental technique called flow cytometry. When it became clear that AIDS was caused by a progressive depletion of CD4 lymphocytes, a central cell of the immune system, Hoxie's research took a different direction. He recalls, "We were the only lab in Philadelphia that could measure CD4 cells. As the work came out, I began to be asked by people, 'Can you do the AIDS test?' I basically told them, 'It's not an AIDS test, but yes, I can measure your CD4 cells.'"[5] Hoxie's hematology clinic began to be visited by gay men who either had AIDS or who had been exposed to somebody with AIDS and were concerned they were at risk and therefore wanted their CD4 cell levels measured. Hoxie became active in working with community groups in Philadelphia who were trying to understand this new disease.

Hoxie credits Cooper for allowing him to pursue this line of research: "Buz saw that this was a problem that involved hematology. AIDS was a new disease and an emerging pandemic. . . . Buz allowed me to look into this problem and encouraged me to attend the first meetings on AIDS that were focused on identifying the cause. Critical to my efforts, he allowed me to hire two technicians while I was still a fellow." Hoxie collected and stored blood specimens from patients with AIDS who were treated at Penn. He provided blood from one of the first Philadelphia patients diagnosed with AIDS to NIH virologist Robert Gallo. From this sample, Gallo isolated one of three viral isolates, later called human immunodeficiency-1 (HIV-1), that were reported in a landmark publication in 1984 in the journal *Science*, showing that this virus was the cause of AIDS.[6] Hoxie dedicated his career at Penn to understanding HIV and how it interacts with CD4 cells and causes disease. In 1998, he established the NIH-funded Penn Center for AIDS Research and served as its Director until 2015.

DuPont Guerry IV trained in internal medicine at Boston City Hospital where his mentors were the hematologists Jim Jandl and Buz Cooper. He recalled, "I fell in love with hematology there and also saw the deep connection between the science of hematology and hematology in the clinic."[7] Once Cooper became Division Chief at Penn, he called Guerry and offered him a position in the fellowship program. As a fellow, Guerry worked in Cooper's laboratory, studying the interaction of red blood cells and macrophages in spherocytic hemolytic anemias.[8] In 1975, he joined the Division to continue bench research in hematology. His career, like Hoxie's, would soon take a radical turn.

In the 1960s and 1970s, Wallace H. Clark Jr., a Harvard dermatopathologist, gained fame for his research into melanocyte biology and melanoma tumorigenesis. His seminal *New England Journal of Medicine* article, "The Clinical Diagnosis, Classification and Histogenic Concepts of the Early Stages of Cutaneous Malignant Melanoma," established the first classification system for melanoma.[9] In 1978, Clark was recruited to the University of Pennsylvania to continue his remarkable career. Cooper brokered a collaboration between Clark and Hilary Koprowski at the Wistar Institute to establish a program to comprehensively study melanoma with the tools of laboratory, clinical, and population science. Clark established Penn's multidisciplinary Pigmented Lesion Clinic where patients with atypical moles and melanoma were evaluated and managed, and Koprowski led studies initially on diagnostic and therapeutic monoclonal antibodies. This clinic-to-lab-to-clinic effort is still funded by an NIH program project.

Cooper had recognized that melanoma represented a potentially fresh field of investigation and Clark would be an outstanding mentor for one of his junior faculty. Guerry recalls that Cooper called him into his office one day: "Buz said, 'Boy, have I got an opportunity for you. This is not only going to solve a cancer, but it's surely going to be a metaphor for the rest of cancer. The name of the disease is melanoma.' I said, 'No.' He said, 'Think about it.'" So Guerry did. He met with Clark and Koprowski and learned more about the exciting research studies and community that he could join. He decided that melanoma was going to be his field and never looked back.

Guerry's research interests were extensive and included biostatistical modeling of melanoma risk and prognosis, the genetics and biology of melanoma susceptibility, and the immunobiology of melanoma. He saw patients weekly in Penn's Pigmented Lesion Clinic. When I was a first-year fellow rotating through this clinic, he taught me how to differentiate atypical nevi, a marker for melanoma risk, from normal moles. He served as Program Leader for the Melanoma Program, a program of Penn's Cancer Center Support Grant (CCSG) since 1978. Despite his melanoma focus, he continued to attend on the hematology consultation service. In 1999, he was named Director of the Division's Hematology/ Oncology fellowship program, a position he held until his retirement in 2009. I asked him what accomplishment of his distinguished career he was most proud of. "From a career and job satisfaction perspective, I probably think that to pick the one thing that was the very best would be my ten years as the Fellowship Director." In recognition of his lifelong commitment to mentoring fellows and junior faculty, the Division established the DuPont Guerry Award for Outstanding Mentorship, which is given yearly to Hematology/Oncology faculty members "who demonstrate exceptional dedication to mentoring and training the next generation of leaders."

In 1979, Douglas Cines joined the Division after completing his Hematology/Oncology fellowship at Penn. As a fellow, he worked closely with Alan Schreiber, an expert in the immunological basis of hematologic disease. Early in his career, Cines, along with Schreiber, added to our understanding of the pathophysiology of immune thrombocytopenic purpura and developed assays for diagnosis of this disease.[10] One of his seminal contributions was delineating the mechanism of heparin-induced thrombocytopenia (HIT). Heparin is frequently used to prevent and treat vascular thrombosis. In up to 0.8 percent of patients receiving heparin, the platelet count decreases and the patient paradoxically is at heightened risk of further thrombosis. HIT is a major cause of morbidity, especially for hospitalized patients. Cines was among the first to explain the immunological mechanism of HIT, reported in 1980 in the *New England Journal of Medicine*.[11] He also helped to develop the platelet ^{14}C-serotonin release functional assay, which is still used to diagnose HIT. Cines and others subsequently demonstrated that HIT is caused by platelet-, endothelial-, and monocyte-activating antibodies that target macromolecular complexes of platelet factor 4 (PF4) and heparin. This led to the development of the anti-PF4/heparin ELISA immunological assay, which has a positive result in nearly 100 percent of patients with HIT.[12] More recently, Cines has partnered with Adam Cuker, a clinical hematologist and translational researcher in our Division, to define and delineate diagnostic and treatment approaches for HIT.[13] In addition to running his research laboratory, Cines served as Director of the Coagulation Laboratory at HUP for over twenty-five years.

After completing his MD and PhD in biochemistry at Case Western Reserve University, where he also trained in internal medicine, Lawrence "Skip" Brass came to Penn as a Hematology/Oncology fellow and subsequently joined the faculty. Brass credits Cooper for his recruitment to Penn. He also recalls his early years on the faculty with Shattil as his mentor. "I started working in platelet biology and became interested in calcium transport into platelets. It turns out that changes in the cytosol calcium concentration of the platelets are critical for platelet activation. Sandy was already interested in the integrin αIIbβ3, then known as glycoprotein IIb/IIIa. We started studying things where our interests overlapped. It turned out that the presence or absence of the integrin αIIbβ3 in platelets in patients with Glanzmann's thrombasthenia influenced calcium transport. Also, it turns out that αIIb, one of the subunits of the integrin, is a calcium binding protein."[14] Brass's ongoing research makes extensive use of genetically engineered mouse models and systems biology approaches to further understand the process of thrombosis and the role of platelet calcium transport.

In addition to his laboratory investigation, Brass has played an important role in the training of physician-scientists at Penn. From 2004 to 2007, he served as Vice Chair for Research in the Department of Medicine. He also served as Associate Dean for Combined Degree and Physician Scholars Programs and as Director of Penn's Medical Scientist Training Program. He has been active at the national level in the development of training programs for physician-scientists and has served as President of the National Association of MD-PhD Programs and Chair of the AAMC GREAT (Association of American Medical Colleges Group on Graduate Research, Education, and Training) section on MD-PhD training, and was a member of the NIH Physician-Scientist Workforce advisory group in 2013–2014. In addition, Brass attends regularly on the Hematology consultation service at HUP.

As the fundamental research of the Division continued to grow, John Glick needed help with the ever-expanding volume of patients with cancer who were coming to Penn. He recalled that he repeatedly asked Cooper to hire a second fellowship-trained medical oncologist. Since they were neighbors, he drove into work every day with Cooper and used this time for mentorship and guidance and to plead his case. "Driving with Buz was the most terrifying thing in the world. He was a scary driver. I'd be beating my head, 'Drive slower. Please hire another oncologist, I'm dying here.' He'd drive faster."[15] Finally, in 1980, Cooper acquiesced, and Glick recruited Daniel Haller.

Haller trained in internal medicine and medical oncology at Georgetown University and then was a senior investigator and Head of the Medicine Section of the Clinical Investigations Branch of the NCI, where he coordinated cooperative group activities, including the Eastern Cooperative Oncology Group (ECOG) and the GI Tumor Study Group, which performed important trials in gastrointestinal cancer for more than a decade. When Glick called Phil Schein and Franco Muggia at Georgetown looking for names, Haller was at the top of the list. Glick and Cooper offered Haller the position and encouraged him to come as soon as possible. Haller recalled, "I realized they were desperate. We were starting to see more and more new patients. It was Peter [Cassileth], John [Glick], Jane [Alavi], and me. John kept pushing my start date up and up, then I realized why. Because nobody ever had a vacation. When I came, John took all of August off, Peter took all of August off, so it was Jane and me and that was it. We had six exam rooms, two chemo chairs, and one chair to do transfusions."[16]

Haller had a remarkable career in the Division. He had a busy outpatient practice, where he initially did general medical oncology but later focused on gastrointestinal (GI) oncology, earning himself a national and international reputation. He rose through the ranks at Penn and was eventually named as the first chair holder of the Deenie Greitzer and Daniel G. Haller, M.D. Associate Professorship in Gastrointestinal Medical Oncology. He was director of the Hematology/Oncology clinic, and as the clinical volume increased, he orchestrated the moves to larger clinic and infusion spaces on the sixth and later sixteenth floors of the Penn Tower Hotel. Haller was an excellent teacher and was one of my primary mentors early in my career at Penn. He served for years as the GI Committee Chair for the ECOG, now called ECOG-ACRIN (American College of Radiology Imaging Network), and Co-Chair of the GI Intergroup, which coordinated all GI clinical research among the cooperative groups.

One of Haller's important research achievements was the development of adjuvant chemotherapy for colorectal cancer. Adjuvant chemotherapy is given after definitive surgery to eradicate any micrometastases that could result in future disease progression and metastasis. In breast cancer, the benefits of adjuvant chemotherapy were unequivocal. While the primary treatment for colorectal cancer was and continues to be surgery, GI oncologists decided to test the concept of adjuvant chemotherapy. At the time, the primary chemotherapy drug was 5-fluorouracil (5-FU). Haller was an important contributor to the national intergroup trial that first demonstrated that adjuvant 5-FU and levamisole decreased the risk of death by a third compared to surgery alone in patients with node-positive colon cancer.[17] He subsequently led a series of important adjuvant colorectal cancer trials to refine this treatment approach. He led a trial demonstrating that six to eight months of adjuvant 5-FU/leucovorin was as efficacious as twelve months of 5-FU/levamisole.[18] He also led a trial comparing the oral chemotherapy regimen capecitabine plus oxaliplatin (XELOX) to standard 5-FU/leucovorin in the adjuvant setting, demonstrating that XELOX was another option for these patients.[19] These studies were important in defining the standards of care for the adjuvant therapy of colorectal cancer.

Haller also had critical and organizational skills that suited him well as an editor. For many years, he was Associate Editor at the *Annals of Internal Medicine* and Editor in Chief of Physician Data Query (PDQ), the NCI's cancer information database. In

2000, Glick encouraged Haller to apply for the position of Editor in Chief of the prestigious *Journal of Clinical Oncology (JCO)*. From 2001 to 2011, Haller was Editor in Chief of *JCO* (per the American Society of Clinical Oncology [ASCO] bylaws, the position is limited to two 5-year terms). Among other accomplishments, he shepherded the journal through the transition from paper to electronic media. Under his leadership, the journal's impact factor increased significantly. He is currently Deputy Editor of *Annals of Oncology*, the journal of the European Society for Medical Oncology. In 2011, ASCO presented him with a Special Recognition Award for his service to the organization. When Haller became Emeritus Professor in 2012, the endowed chair he held was renamed in his honor. The Deenie Greitzer and Daniel G. Haller, MD Associate Professorship in Gastrointestinal Medical Oncology is currently held by Penn GI oncologist Ursina Teitelbaum. She is an outstanding medical oncologist who is Clinical Director of the Penn Pancreatic Cancer Research Center.

Like much of medicine in the early 1970s, the Division of Hematology/Oncology was predominantly male. However, two notable women were members of the early faculty. Jane Alavi trained in hematology at Penn in 1969–1970. On completing her fellowship, she became a hematologist at Philadelphia General Hospital (PGH). PGH was the public hospital of Philadelphia akin to Bellevue Hospital in New York City and Boston City Hospital. Although trained as a hematologist, Alavi by necessity saw oncology patients at PGH. She recalled, "I taught myself medical oncology. I had no training. No one taught me anything, I just did it myself. We all learned on the job. I took and passed the first medical oncology boards."[20] Glick was at Cooper's home having coffee when Cooper heard the news on the radio that PGH was closing. Cooper jumped up, got on the phone, and immediately offered Alavi a job at HUP. She practiced both hematology and medical oncology and became interested in clinical research. In fact, she conducted the first randomized trial of white blood cell transfusions to prevent infections in patients with leukemia, a study that was published in the *New England Journal of Medicine*.[21]

Early in her career, Alavi was asked by Cooper to perform Hematology/Oncology outreach in Hazleton, a town in the Pocono Mountains of Pennsylvania. She recalled,

> After I started on the faculty here, doctors in Hazleton contacted Penn and set up some type of a cooperative arrangement and since they did not have oncologists, they wanted a hematologist/oncologist to help them out. The solution to this was to send me to Hazleton one day every two weeks. This went on for at least a year, maybe two years. I'd drive early in the morning over the mountains down into Hazleton, and I'd get there about 9:00 or 9:30 to run a clinic at Saint Joseph's Hospital. The nurse was wonderful. She had this little clinic for me, and the patients would line up. They were just wonderful. Salt of the earth kind of people. They would bring you gifts and bake things for you. I saw anemias, I saw metastasized cancers, I did bone marrows. I did everything myself, I gave chemotherapy myself. I did that in the morning, and then sometime in the afternoon I went over to the other hospital, Hazleton General, for inpatient consultations. Then I drove home.

Alavi spent her entire career at Penn and continued to be an active learner and teacher. During the latter part of her career, she became the Division's primary neuro-oncologist, becoming an expert at treating patients with brain tumors. She was principal investigator of an R01 research grant to develop adenovirus-based gene therapy for patients with refractory brain tumors. In 2003, Alavi retired from the Division and currently spends much of her time volunteering at the Morris Arboretum of the University of Pennsylvania.

When Janet Abrahm was a medical student at the University of California at San Francisco, she worked with Shattil, who was a U.S. Public Health Service officer at the time. She trained in internal medicine at Massachusetts General Hospital, and after a year back at UC San Francisco as Chief Resident, she came to Penn for a fellowship in Hematology/Oncology (1977 to 1980). She recalled, "The reason I did it was because I was following Sandy."[22] Cooper invited her to join the faculty after her fellow-ship, with a focus on hematopoiesis (the production of blood cells) research. She spent most of her time at the Veterans Hospital of Philadelphia where she had funding. "A year after I went over, the person who was there decided to leave. I became the Chief of Hematology/Oncology." She remained there as Division Chief and then was Chair of Medicine until 1997.

Over time, Abrahm's focus switched from fundamental hema-topoiesis research to clinical interests, such as pain management and palliative care. In 1992, she undertook a sabbatical at Memo-rial Sloan Kettering Cancer Center in New York City, where she worked with giants in the field of palliative care and pain manage-ment, such as Kathy Foley. From 1997 to 1999, she was funded by the Project on Death in America as a faculty scholar with the mis-sion to understand and transform the experience of dying through initiatives in research and scholarship. The Project on Death was established in 1994 by the Open Society Institute, a nonprofit foundation started by philanthropist George Soros.[23] These years were transformational for Abrahm, who devoted the remainder of her career to palliative care. She established a palliative care fellowship at Penn and was Medical Director of Wissahickon Hospice at Penn from 1998 to 2000. In 2001, she was recruited to Harvard, where she became Chief of the Division of Adult Palliative Care and where she remains as Professor of Medicine. Her book *A Physician's Guide to Pain and Symptom Management in Cancer Patients* is considered a classic.

FIVE

Change in Leadership

In 1985, Buz Cooper left Penn to become Dean of the Medical School at the Medical College of Wisconsin. His departure left unfilled two important leadership positions: Chief of the Hematology/Oncology Division and Director of the University of Pennsylvania Cancer Center. Cooper's protégé, Sandy Shattil, was a logical choice for Chief of the Division of Hematology/Oncology. He was recognized as an outstanding platelet biologist and clinical hematologist. Shattil recalled, "At that time, the department chair, Larry Earley, asked me to take over the division, which I did for about six or seven years."[1] During his tenure as Division Chief, Shattil focused on growing the bench research program.

Charles Abrams transferred to Penn from Temple during his internal medicine residency. He recalled doing an elective on the Hematology consultation service with Shattil and subsequently working in Shattil's laboratory. "He was full of energy. There was nothing that he saw that he didn't want to look up and explore more. He was always rigorous. But in the end, you felt like the patients got good care because of this stern father figure and assertive physician. Then, as a senior resident, I pulled all of my elective time together for a five-month block and worked in Sandy's lab and started doing platelet research."[2] Abrams completed his Hematology/Oncology fellowship in 1991 and then joined the faculty, just as his mentor Shattil was leaving the Division.

Fortunately, Shattil's colleague Skip Brass took Abrams under his wing: "Skip said, 'You and I are going to have joint lab meetings. You and your one technician in my lab, we're going to get together every Wednesday morning. We're going to present our experiments to each other, and we're going to talk science and what we should be doing next.'" The approach worked, as Abrams has had a prolific research career focused on understanding the biochemistry of phospholipid signaling in platelets and T cells. He presently is the Francis C. Wood Professor of Medicine, Vice Chair of Medicine for Research, and Chief Scientific Officer of the Perelman School of Medicine.

In 1990, Shattil recruited Alan Gewirtz to the Division from Temple University. Gewirtz's research focus was in developing novel therapeutics for leukemia, including pioneering "anti-sense" therapy with interfering RNA oligonucleotides. Targeting the *c-myb* proto-oncogene, he and my co-fellow Selina Luger performed a pilot trial of *c-myb* anti-sense therapy in patients with refractory leukemia.[3] Gewirtz became the C. Willard Robinson Professor of Hematology-Oncology and in 1998 was named Director of the Cancer Center's Hematologic Malignancy Program. He was an avid pilot and was even funded by NASA to study hematopoiesis in outer space. Sadly, Gewirtz died of advanced lung cancer on November 17, 2010. In a tribute to his colleague, Abrams wrote,

"More important than Alan's outstanding career and his scientific contributions, is the way in which he led his life. He had that perfect and enviable balance, which allowed him to excel without taking himself or life too seriously. He would not hesitate to debate with you, while Sparky, his dog, dutifully remained by his side. Not only was he brilliant and indefatigable, he was also caring, funny, and kind. He had an endless zest for life and learning. Alan was that bright light that will forever live on in the hearts of all those around the world whom he touched."[4]

Other key research faculty recruited by Shattil included Keith McCrae who worked closely with Douglas Cines and then at the Cleveland Clinic; J. Eric Russell who is an Associate Professor of Medicine in the Division with a focus on the control and function of embryonic hemoglobin genes; William Lee, a molecular biologist who studied the *c-myc* oncogene in cancer progression as well as angiogenesis and retired in 2015; and Elwyn Loh, who studied T cell gene rearrangement in B cell malignancies and was on the faculty for ten years until he left in 1999 to join the pharmaceutical industry.

———

In 1985, John Glick succeeded Cooper as Director of the University of Pennsylvania Cancer Center. Under the next twenty-one years of his leadership, the center grew significantly in size, funding, and stature. "Building the Abramson Cancer Center from a fledgling cancer organization to one of the best-known and best-funded cancer centers in the world was a singular accomplishment that I'm very proud of," Glick said. "We went from having approximately a hundred members to having more than three hundred members, and from having $10 million per year in external grants to having $175 million per year in grants. We went on to be one of the top cancer centers in the country."[5] Glick served as Cancer Center Director until 2006, making him at the time the longest-serving Director of an NCI-designated comprehensive cancer center.[6] As principal investigator of the Cancer Center Support Grant, Glick successfully achieved the competitive renewal of this grant four times, increasing total yearly CCSG funding from $2 million to $7.5 million.

Glick focused on the expansion of the medical oncology program. Over the next several years, he recruited a number of new clinical faculty members. The first was Donna Glover, who had trained at Penn in Hematology/Oncology and focused her clinical practice on breast cancer, melanoma, and lung cancer as well as clinical trials. She was a lead investigator in the development of the radio- and chemo-protectant WR2721 that was subsequently approved by the FDA.[7] In 1990, Glover left the Division to become chief of Hematology/Oncology at Presbyterian Medical Center and then subsequently went into private practice. She died in 2019.

Kevin Fox completed medical school and an internal medicine residency at Johns Hopkins. During his second year of residency he decided to focus on hematology/oncology. He recalled, "As interns, we rotated through the oncology center, and what I was struck by was the stark contrast between general medicine in a hospital and oncology medicine in a hospital. Everybody's diagnosis was firm. Everybody's therapeutic plan was firm. Everything was protocol-driven. Care standards were adhered to rigidly. And I was sort of caught up in a thrall of this entity, which seemed organized and enthusiastic and everything was new. A few months of inpatient oncology convinced me that this was something I was interested in."[8]

Fox came to Penn for Hematology/Oncology fellowship training in 1984. As a second- and third-year fellow, he worked closely with Glick. Fox told me, "With his appointment as Cancer Center Director, John created this entity which was known as 'Glick's fellow' in which an upper-year fellow worked closely with him. This was essentially a full-time job. And so that became my existence as a fellow. I helped John take care of his patients and had a lot of exposure to breast cancer and lymphoma. At that time, the clinical investigation that was being done in the Division was pretty much limited to clinical trials of the substance called WR2721, which was being tested as a chemo-protectant. My other job was to help with those clinical trials." In 1988, Fox joined the Division as an Assistant Professor of Medicine. From the start, he proved himself to be a superb clinical medical oncologist. He developed a large clinical practice, initially seeing patients with breast cancer and lymphoma and later focusing his practice exclusively on breast cancer.

Soon after Glick became Cancer Center Director in 1985, he chaired the pivotal NCI Consensus Conference on the adjuvant treatment of breast cancer. The results of this conference changed the standard of care for patients with early breast cancer and were published in the *Journal of the American Medical Association*.[9] Increasingly, medical oncologists played an important and expanding role in the management of all patients with breast cancer. Fox reflected on how breast cancer oncology evolved over the years from when he first joined the faculty. "In a developed country where mammographic screening is widely available, most women will be diagnosed with early-stage breast cancer. Before 1989, oncologists generally were asked only to see patients who had positive axillary lymph nodes at the time of their breast surgery. Those patients were treated with postoperative therapy. The patients with negative lymph nodes were not felt to be appropriate candidates for postoperative therapy, and we never saw them. For those patients receiving postoperative therapy, systemic chemotherapy was the predominant intervention. Endocrine therapy was something of a novelty at that time. All of that changed rather abruptly in 1989. That's when all the clinical trials in node-negative women were published and legitimized treatment of those women as well. In 1989, the number of women seeking consultation for postoperative therapy doubled. At the same time, the widespread use of endocrine therapy for estrogen receptor–positive women became the care standard. The use of chemotherapy became more restricted, and that's how things would go for the next fifteen years. Then in 2005, the advent of genomic testing in patients with estrogen receptor–positive, lymph node–negative breast cancer began to identify groups of women for whom chemotherapy was not needed. Now years later, the struggle is whether to apply those same rules to node-positive patients."

By all measures, Fox is a master clinician. He has seen it all and always puts the patient's interests first. In 2002, he was awarded the I. S. Ravdin Master Clinician Award and is a founding member of Penn Medicine's Academy of Master Clinicians, which was conceived and created by Glick in 2013. Like many members of the Hematology/Oncology faculty, Fox has spent his career at Penn. He thinks this is largely a result of loyalty. He stated, "I think loyalty here is at several levels. Loyalty to the division is enormous. We see ourselves first as members of the Division; second, as members of the Department of Medicine; third, as members of the University of Pennsylvania Health System. Maybe in retrospect, that's the greatest success of the Division. Making people feel the loyalty to the Division first and foremost and oblivious to everything else."

When he was a fourth-year Penn medical student, Edward Stadtmauer greatly enjoyed his elective in hematology. Alan Schreiber was his attending, and Skip Brass was the fellow on the service. During his internal medicine residency at Albert Einstein Medical Center in the Bronx, Stadtmauer worked closely with the Head of Hematology, Christine Laurence. He knew he wanted to pursue a career in hematology/oncology. He was accepted in the Memorial Sloan Kettering fellowship and called Schreiber to tell him the great news. Schreiber convinced him to come to Penn to train instead.[10]

Stadtmauer started his fellowship in 1986. His first rotation was on the ten-bed oncology unit on the seventh floor of the Silverstein Pavilion, which was mainly treating leukemia. As a fellow, he worked closely with Peter Cassileth, a nationally recognized leukemia specialist. Stadtmauer recalled, "I went with Peter because I was interested in the leukemia stuff. My proposal to him was, we don't have a bone marrow transplant program and I think we need a bone marrow transplant program." Stadtmauer joined the faculty in 1989 and worked with Cassileth to create an autologous bone marrow transplant program. With autologous transplantation, a patient who had bone marrow harvested underwent high-dose myeloablative chemotherapy followed by reinfusion of the patient's own bone marrow cells. The reinfused marrow "rescued" the patient from the potentially life-threatening complications of high-dose chemotherapy. At the time, autologous transplantation was being evaluated in many types of cancer, both hematologic (for example, relapsed or refractory lymphoma) and solid tumors (for example, metastatic breast cancer). When Cassileth left Penn in 1992 to become Chief of the Division of Hematology/Oncology at the University of Miami,

Stadtmauer became the most senior member of the Division focusing on hematologic malignancies and autologous bone marrow transplantation.

In the 1990s, high-dose chemotherapy with autologous transplantation was being touted as a breakthrough for women with metastatic breast cancer. The rationale behind high-dose chemotherapy for a disease such as metastatic breast cancer was that "more is better." Some investigators reported promising results from this approach in phase I and II trials. Hence, high-dose chemotherapy with autologous transplantation was widely being used to treat women with metastatic breast cancer, although there was no randomized trial comparing this approach to standard-dose chemotherapy. The importance of such a trial cannot be overstated, since high-dose therapy was associated with increased toxicity and increased cost compared to conventional chemotherapy. It would only be worth doing if survival were prolonged. Glick organized a consortium called the Philadelphia Bone Marrow Transplant Group and together with Stadtmauer designed the PBT-1 randomized trial that compared high-dose chemotherapy with conventional-dose chemotherapy in patients with metastatic breast cancer. Glick obtained a grant from U.S. Healthcare to fund this trial, which subsequently expanded to include the Mayo Clinic, Johns Hopkins, and ECOG.

At the Plenary Session of the 1999 ASCO meeting, Stadtmauer presented the results of PBT-1. The trial showed no evidence that high-dose chemotherapy improved survival in patients with metastatic breast cancer. In his presentation, Stadtmauer concluded, "This largest randomized trial of bone marrow transplant in metastatic breast cancer demonstrates no improvement in overall survival with transplant, no improvement in time to progression or progression-free survival with transplant, no substantial difference in lethal toxicity. Non-lethal serious toxicities were greater in the transplant arm, particularly hematologic, infection, nausea and diarrhea. Obviously, from the survival curves, these results will not change with more follow-up in this study."[11] Glick and Stadtmauer's PBT-1 trial was the definitive randomized trial to demonstrate that high-dose chemotherapy resulted in no survival advantage compared to conventional-dose therapy in patients with metastatic breast cancer. Although its results were disappointing, this trial was an important achievement because women with metastatic breast cancer would no longer be subjected to the toxicity and cost of unnecessary high-dose chemotherapy. Kevin Fox believes that PBT-1 is "one of the greatest achievements of this Division." This practice-changing trial was subsequently published in the *New England Journal of Medicine*, with Stadtmauer as first author and Glick as senior author.[12]

Stadtmauer has spent his career at Penn and is Section Chief for Hematologic Malignancies. He has subsequently focused much of his effort on building the multiple myeloma program. He was very involved in the development of autologous transplant for this disease. More recently, he has been at the forefront in the development of novel agents for myeloma. He recently published in *Science* the first-in-human, phase I clinical trial designed to test the safety and feasibility of multiplex CRISPR-Cas9 gene editing of T cells from patients with advanced, refractory cancer including myeloma.[13] In 2017, he was named as the first endowed chair holder of the Roseman, Tarte, Harrow, and Shaffer Families' President's Distinguished Professorship. When I asked him among his many accomplishments what he is most proud of, he stated, "You know what I'm most proud of? I'm very proud of our progeny and our colleagues. I feel prouder every time we go to the ASCO meet-

ing or the ASH [American Society of Hematology] meeting."
Every year, Stadtmauer puts together for the Division detailed
summaries of what Penn investigators will present at the annual
ASH and ASCO meetings. "Maybe that's also a part of it, right?
Why we stay here is that somehow this place has been magical
enough to make this all happen."

When Lynn Schuchter was a third-year medical oncology fellow at Johns Hopkins, she interviewed at several major centers for
a faculty position. She had spent her fellowship focused on developing novel treatment approaches to melanoma. She had an interest in biological response modifiers and was studying a compound
called bryostatin. Although she had an offer in hand from the
University of North Carolina at Chapel Hill, she had one more
institution to visit. She recalls her first visit to Penn: "I came and
gave a talk on melanoma immunotherapy and a clinical trial I was
doing. I had a fantastic day visiting. DuPont [Guerry] was amazing. Wally Clark interviewed me, and I remember thinking that
I knew so much, coming from Hopkins. I interviewed with him,
and it was like I didn't know anything. He was just light years
ahead. I was very impressed with my first visit."[14] She recognized
that there was a great opportunity at Penn with Guerry and Clark
as mentors, the Pigmented Lesion Clinic as a clinical and research
hub, and very little going on in the Division at the time with
respect to developmental therapeutics for melanoma. Glick and
Shattil offered her a position.

She had one concern, though. Although Schuchter was single,
she knew she ultimately wanted a family and realized that she had
never discussed the Division's maternity leave policy. So she made
a special trip back to Penn to meet with Glick and Shattil to have
the policy clearly explained. She recalled, "They were totally
flummoxed. I remember John had a credenza behind him, and

he's trying to find a policy and there is no policy. Basically, he says, 'There is no policy but whatever you want, we'll figure it out.' They were definitely not comfortable, but they communicated that they would be flexible." Despite this one lingering concern, Schuchter accepted the position and began her career at Penn in July 1989.

Initially, Schuchter had three days each week where she cared for outpatients with melanoma, as well as with lymphoma and breast cancer. She also attended in Pigmented Lesion Clinic weekly, where dermatologists and multiple other specialists evaluated patients with pigmented skin lesions. "We all participated, surgeons, medical oncologists, dermatologists. That is the culture that was evident thirty years ago." Using the melanoma database, she developed a prognostic model that more accurately predicted ten-year survival in primary melanoma than using tumor thickness alone.[15] She also performed investigator-initiated clinical trials. One early trial that she did with the dermatologist Allan Halpern deserves mention because of its innovative trial design. Schuchter took patients with dysplastic nevi syndrome, a condition in which patients have atypical-appearing moles and are at risk for developing malignant melanoma, and painted half of each patients back with topical tretinoin, a vitamin A analogue, using the unpainted half of the patient's back as the control. With use of tretinoin, dysplastic nevi regressed and biopsies of nevi from the tretinoin treatment demonstrated much less atypia than the untreated nevi.[16] Schuchter also performed clinical trials of novel agents in patients with metastatic melanoma, a field in which she would rapidly become a national expert.

Schuchter reflected on Guerry's mentorship, which was a key to her success. "Extraordinary. Very supportive. I knew very few people in Philadelphia. I became very close to his family and his children. He was like a friend and a mentor and still is a close friend and a mentor. I still have him read and edit things that I write." Early on, Glick also involved Schuchter in the administration of the Cancer Center's clinical trials program, naming her Director of the Clinical Research Unit. She also would write the Cancer Center's institutional Data and Safety Monitoring Plan. She has continued her administrative leadership throughout her career, serving as Program Leader for the Melanoma Program, and ultimately she became Associate Director for Clinical Research at the Cancer Center. From the start, Schuchter was very involved

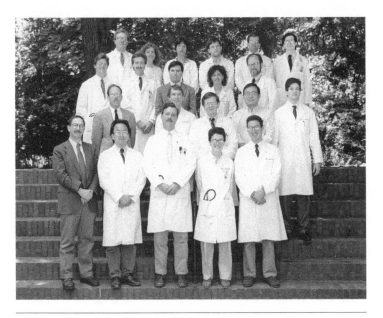

Figure 2. Division, 1990. Division Chief Sanford "Sandy" Shattil is in the front row, first from left.

in ASCO, serving through the years in several important leadership positions.

_____

This was the state of the Division of Hematology/Oncology when I arrived for my first day of fellowship training in July 1990: a very strong bench research program in benign hematology and a small but outstanding medical oncology program that excelled in clinical care and had a strong presence in cooperative group trials and a developing investigator-initiated clinical trials program.

SIX

Fellowship

Present at orientation on my first day of fellowship in July 1990 were three other tyros: Selina Luger, who would later become Director of the Leukemia service at the Hospital of the University of Pennsylvania; Will Luginbuhl, who joined an outstanding private practice group in West Chester, Pennsylvania; and Ralph Vassallo, who later would become Chief Medical Officer of the American Red Cross Blood Service–East Division. We met in a small conference room on Silverstein 7 where Sandy Shattil reviewed for us what the year would entail and where we also met with the exiting first-year fellows, who enthusiastically greeted us with relieved looks on their faces.

The first year of our fellowship would be entirely clinical. We would rotate through the various services of the Division: Inpatient Oncology Unit, Hematology consultation service, and Medical Oncology consultation service. We also would have a hematology/oncology clinic where we saw outpatients with an assigned faculty mentor.

As promised, it was a very demanding year, and like most groups placed into challenging settings, we became a close team, helping each other through the year. My first rotation was the Inpatient Oncology Unit, a ten-bed unit housed on Silverstein 7. This was largely a leukemia unit, although other patients were admitted there for a variety of inpatient chemotherapy regimens, such as combination chemotherapy for testicular cancer or lymphoma. My assigned attending was James Hoxie, then deeply involved in HIV laboratory research. He was a very thoughtful, detail-oriented attending who was a master at treating acute leukemia. I was amazed at his devotion to patients and his ability to recall minor details about all the patients on our service. He was a demanding but fair attending. I worked hard to live up to his high expectations.

During this time, I had a young patient with acute promyelocytic leukemia (APML). She was a mother of two with a steadfast husband. One of the unique aspects of patients with APML is their propensity to have severe bleeding and/or clotting complications because of leukemia-related disseminated intravascular coagulation (DIC). When induction chemotherapy was initiated and tumor cells were killed, this DIC would often get so out of control that life-threatening complications developed. We would paradoxically start these patients on the anticoagulant heparin to reverse the DIC. And as one might expect, the clinical course of these patients was often complicated. Tragically, my patient suffered an intracerebral hemorrhage and never made it out of the hospital.

As an aside, a major advance for patients with APML was the development of all-trans retinoic acid (ATRA). Interestingly,

ATRA was initially developed by Alfred Kligman of Penn Dermatology as a treatment for acne.[1] However, the drug was later demonstrated to cause differentiation of white blood cells, which was therapeutically taken advantage of in treating APML.[2] With ATRA, patients with APML could be "eased" into remission, avoiding much of the DIC associated with induction chemotherapy for this disease. Unfortunately, ATRA would not come into widespread use for APML until later that decade. After a couple of month-long rotations in the Inpatient Oncology Unit, where I witnessed several deaths of young patients undergoing induction chemotherapy for acute leukemia, I was certain of one thing: I did not want to be a leukemia specialist.

The Hematology consultation service was very different. I came to fellowship anticipating a career in hematology. On this consult service, we were asked to see very complicated patients, often those who had been in the intensive care unit for weeks. The most common reason for the consult was thrombocytopenia (a decreased platelet count). The possible causes of this thrombocytopenia were myriad, and it often took hours of poring over volumes of medical records to narrow these for a particular patient. Shattil was my attending for one of these rotations. Although largely laboratory focused, he was an extraordinary and demanding clinician. He required that we manually perform blood smears on every consultation, and we would then discuss the case at the multiheaded microscope in what came to be known as the "fellow's room" located outside of the Inpatient Unit on Silverstein 7. Not uncommonly, Shattil would take one look at my smear and get up and leave. "Call me when you have a decent smear for me to look at." As fellows, we also performed and then stained our bone marrow aspirations. It was remarkably satisfying that in a matter of an hour or so, one could extract bone marrow, review it, and

come up with an explanation for why a patient had thrombocytopenia or anemia.

As the fellow on the Hematology consultation service, I was
also responsible for putting together case presentations for the
Hematology conference that met every Friday afternoon. This is
the same conference started by Buz Cooper that John Glick, on
his first visit, referred to as a "lunatic asylum." Hematology conference was a highly stressful experience for fellows, because not
only did you need to identify interesting cases, preferably with a
firm diagnosis, but you had to show blood and bone marrow smears
to the group and be fully able to discuss the scientific basis of the
diseases that you presented. The attending hematologists would
endlessly argue with each other about the cases. One of my strate-
gies was to present the case and then let the attendings fight it out
while I ducked for cover. I remember a sense of profound relief
when the conference ended. My co-fellow Vassallo was an absolute master at presenting at these conferences. He would have the
best cases and the most interesting and highest-quality smears,
and would pass around well-researched handouts with tables that
could have been published in a textbook. The rest of us were not so
talented. Although I came to Penn planning to be a hematologist,
the tedium of the consultations and the dread of the weekly conference made me doubt that this was the right career path for me.

However, I greatly enjoyed both my outpatient Oncology clinic
and my rotations on the inpatient Oncology consultation service.
Daniel Haller was my supervising attending for these during that
first year. He was very smart, very funny, and full of medical wis-
dom, teaching me at the bedside oncologic principles that I have
never forgotten. One vivid example: When considering a patient
with rectal cancer, "Never underestimate the misery of an uncon-
trolled pelvic recurrence." On the Oncology consultation service

with Haller, I remember seeing two young men with metastatic testicular cancer. We enrolled both patients in an Eastern Cooperative Oncology Group phase III clinical trial that compared the standard chemotherapy regimen of bleomycin, etoposide, and cisplatin with etoposide, ifosfamide, and cisplatin in patients with poor-prognosis disease. I was amazed as both patients' serum tumor markers rapidly normalized, symptoms rapidly improved, and a large, left-sided neck mass in one of the patients literally melted away in a few days. Both entered durable remissions and never relapsed, cured of a disease that in 1970 would have killed them both. I was hooked: I knew then and there that I wanted to become a medical oncologist.

As first year of my fellowship ended, I recall meeting with Shattil to talk about plans for the next two years, which would be largely research focused. He explained the importance of spending time in the laboratory during this research experience. "The question isn't if you are going into the lab, but whose lab you are going into." Because my career interest was now cancer focused, he suggested that I spend the two years in the laboratory of William M. F. Lee. Lee was a molecular biologist studying the proto-oncogene *myc* and its role in driving tumor cell growth. However, he was branching out into a new line of inquiry in collaboration with DuPont Guerry, who had demonstrated that cells from advanced melanomas failed to present antigen to initiate an immune response. The question was why. Guerry and Lee hypothesized that it was due to a molecular abnormality in the human leukocyte antigen–DR isotope complex caused by a mutation. My project was to prove this was the case.

Some physicians are great in the laboratory. They enjoy asking fundamental questions and setting out to answer them. They may also have "great hands," that is, the ability to perform laboratory experiments with grace and agility. And when an experiment did not work, they find this interesting and are challenged to figure out why. And then there was me. I was not a natural in the laboratory, finding tasks like pouring sequencing gel between two large glass plates nearly impossible. I did not like the pace of laboratory research. And when an experiment did not work, I did not find it interesting, just disappointing and frustrating. It was nothing like treating testicular cancer with chemotherapy, where there was immediate gratification as tumors disappeared over a course of days to weeks. For me, laboratory research was the ultimate deferral of gratification. I started to dread going to the laboratory and became a bit depressed over the prospect of doing this for my life's work. After a year of failed experiments (and broken glassware), I knew that I was not destined to be a laboratory scientist. I remember explaining first to Lee and then to Shattil and Guerry my decision to leave the laboratory after only a year. In retrospect, it was a valuable year in which I learned a lot of science—and a lot about myself.

As a first-year fellow, I interacted with Glick mainly at our weekly Oncology case conference where cases were presented by faculty and fellows and Glick ran the management discussion. I was impressed with his mastery of oncology and sound clinical approach to patients. However, he had a reputation as being a difficult and demanding attending. He was well into his tenure as Director of the University of Pennsylvania Cancer Center and was considered the premier oncologist in Philadelphia for patients with breast cancer and lymphoma. At the end of my first year of fellowship, he called me into his office and invited me to be his fellow for the next two years. While I knew this would be a great opportunity and one I could not pass up, I wondered how I could possibly do this and go into Lee's laboratory. Glick tried to limit my clinical work to one day per week to allow me protected time for my laboratory training, but of course clinical medicine does not always work like that. There were always emergencies to see, urgent phone calls to answer, and chart notes to complete. It became a difficult balance. In fact, I kept a necktie in my laboratory desk drawer so that if Glick called, I would put in on as I was running over to clinic, and then on my way back to the lab remove it and hide it from Lee's knowing eyes.

Despite the demands, I absolutely loved being a "Glick fellow." He was an outstanding teacher and the most detail-oriented clinician I had ever worked with. In his patient charts were his legendary flow sheets, where you could track everything that you needed to know about a patient's clinical course without ever reading a note. I learned to always meticulously update the clinic flow sheets. I saw patients with breast cancer and lymphoma and learned how to give chemotherapy. He taught me about dose modifications, managing toxicity, and how to determine if a patient is benefiting from treatment or not. He also taught me what to do when therapy no longer works, how to manage cancer-related symptoms, and how to help the patient and family during the final stage of the disease. It was a transformative experience that changed the direction of my career.

One afternoon, I was paged to the very familiar "662-6334" and promptly returned the call. Glick instructed me, "Meet me at my office at 5 P.M.; we are going to make a house call." We had a patient who was a prominent Philadelphia stockbroker with an aggressive non-Hodgkin's lymphoma. Despite standard and salvage chemotherapy, he had progressive disease, and it was clear he was not going to survive this cancer. That evening we drove out to his stately home in a beautiful Quaker town in New Jersey. We entered the home and found our patient in bed, uncomfortable and agitated and the family at his bedside. Glick took charge of the situation. He told the family that the patient was in the terminal phase of his illness and that the goal was comfort and a peaceful death. With appropriate medications and home hospice support, he was able to die peacefully a few days later in his home of many decades, with his loving wife and children surrounding him. I realized that cancer medicine was not only about the cure.

As I started my third year of fellowship, I was finishing clinic notes on a Saturday morning when I bumped into Haller, who was sitting on the floor on the sixth floor of Penn Tower, examining patient charts and corresponding clinical trials case report forms from his large Intergroup adjuvant colorectal cancer clinical trial. He asked how I was, and I described my recent laboratory experience and how I felt in some ways like a failure and that I loved clinical oncology but did not know what kind of research I could do. "You should do what we do: clinical trials." He explained to me about the work he was doing through ECOG as a leader in gastrointestinal oncology.

He suggested that I could help him on a pilot clinical trial he was conducting combining 5-FU, leucovorin, and interferon-alfa with radiation for the treatment of locally advanced upper gastrointestinal cancer. I jumped at the opportunity. This pilot trial became my trial. I recruited, evaluated, and treated the patients; collected and analyzed the data; and presented the results in 1993 at the national meeting of the American Association of Cancer Research. I had found a field of research that was interesting and important, and allowed me to do what I was best at: taking care of patients. As my third year of fellowship ended, I now knew what I wanted to be: an academic medical oncologist with a focus on clinical trials in solid tumors.

SEVEN

The 1990s

In 1989, William Kelley was recruited to Penn to become Dean of the School of Medicine and Chief Executive Officer of the Medical Center. As Chair of the Department of Medicine at the University of Michigan, Kelley, a rheumatologist who had made important discoveries related to purine metabolism, built a formidable program, recruiting a world-class research faculty. When he arrived in Philadelphia, Kelley set about establishing the University of Pennsylvania Health System (UPHS), the nation's first fully integrated university health system. He brought Pennsylvania Hospital, Presbyterian Hospital, and Phoenixville Hospital into UPHS. He also acquired many private practice groups throughout the Delaware Valley as a strategy to ensure referral of complex patients into the medical center. Under his leadership, Penn moved from tenth to second in NIH funding, and the School of Medicine improved from tenth to third in the *US News and World Report* ranking of research-oriented medical schools. New research buildings went up. He charged a redesign of the medical school curriculum, and Curriculum 2000 was developed and implemented. It was clear that Kelley was a mover and a shaker and that Penn was changing.

Kelley recruited Edward Holmes, a former trainee, fellow rheumatologist, and close associate to become Chair of the Department of Medicine. Holmes served in this position from 1991 to 1997. As leader of the Department of Medicine, the Chair is responsible for the Division Chiefs who report to him. In 1992, Sandy Shattil began to feel that it was time for a change, both for the Division and for himself. He recalled that "one of the main precipitants to me dropping out as division chief was a disagreement with the department chair at that time over some financial issues."[1] He submitted his resignation to Holmes, who accepted it.

In 1992, Shattil started to focus more on his research program. In 1994, he spent a sabbatical year doing bench research at the Scripps Research Institute in La Jolla, California. Then, coupled with the spectacular scientific environment on the La Jolla Mesa and the jogging weather in San Diego, Shattil moved with his family there and spent the next ten years at Scripps focusing on unraveling molecular aspects of platelet function. In 2004, he was recruited to the University of California at San Diego to serve as Chief of the Division of Hematology/Oncology, and he remains there today as a Distinguished Professor of Medicine. From 2003 to 2007, he served as Editor in Chief of the prestigious hematology journal *Blood*. Reflecting on his years as Division Chief at Penn, Shattil told me, "I don't think of too many downs. I think the main accomplishment during those years was to survive the loss of Buz Cooper and to start growing the Division again, all in a relatively small way compared to the spectacular growth that happened years later."

With Shattil's departure, Holmes asked John Glick and Joel Bennett to serve as interim Division Co-Chiefs, which they did from 1993 to 1995. Glick's focus was medical oncology, the clinical practice, and clinical research, while Bennett's was hematology and bench research. These two senior members of the Division had a very effective partnership. In the spring of 1993, as I was completing my third year of fellowship, my pager went off and it was Glick's office. He wanted to discuss something important and told me to come immediately to his office. I thought it must have to do with one of our patients, but in fact he had me sit down across from his big desk and asked me about my future plans. He told me that the Division needed medical oncologists and that I was an excellent clinician and a hard worker. To my great surprise, he offered me a position as an Assistant Professor of Medicine focusing on gastrointestinal cancer, helping Daniel Haller with the increasing number of these patients. He handed me an offer letter spelling out the details of the position and my starting salary of $72,000. He told me that the terms were not up for negotiation and that I was fortunate to be joining such a great institution. I was thrilled. I signed the letter on the spot and in July 1993, I joined the Division.

These initial years were clinically very busy. I saw patients four days per week, largely patients with gastrointestinal tract malignancies but also patients with genitourinary and breast cancer and lymphoma. I tried to do clinical research as well, although this was largely at nights and on weekends. I also rotated as attending on the inpatient service in one-month blocks, including all four weekends. It was hard work, but I enjoyed it.

As I was well into my third year as a faculty member, I was approached by one of the Penn urologists. "Why is no one in your Division interested in genitourinary cancer?" He was right. The patients with genitourinary (GU) cancer were referred to several of us, but for none of us was it our main focus. I thought about this question for a couple of days. I enjoyed working with Haller and found gastrointestinal cancer interesting. However, I realized that with Haller's national and international reputation, I would never become the Penn gastrointestinal cancer leader. I called my urology colleague and told him I was game to focus on GU cancer. And like that, I became our Division's GU oncologist.

GU oncology includes cancer of the bladder, kidney, prostate, and testis. For the next twelve years, I was the only GU oncologist in the Division. I essentially taught myself GU oncology, but truth be told, at the time treatment options for bladder, kidney, and prostate cancer were rather limited. This is in marked contrast to the present situation where significant progress has been made in developing new agents for these diseases. Testicular cancer was a different story. Significant progress had already been made with treatment for testicular cancer, including the development of curative cisplatin-based chemotherapy for patients with metastatic disease. These were mostly young men, and the stakes were obviously high. I had always enjoyed taking care of patients with testicular cancer, and, as the GU oncologist at Penn, I would be responsible for this group of patients. However, there was no one on campus who was a bona fide expert in the field. As a junior faculty member, when I had a complex testicular cancer case where I frankly did not know what to do, I often turned to someone outside of the institution for guidance. I had on speed-dial two of the giants in testicular cancer: Larry Einhorn at Indiana University and George Bosl at Memorial Sloan Kettering Cancer

Center. To their credit, they always returned my calls and provided invaluable assistance. I am sure that I was one of several fledging testicular cancer providers who turned to them for help. I am indebted to them for their selfless mentorship of a young physician outside of their own institutions.

In 1995, Glick was elected President of the American Society of Clinical Oncology. He called me into his office to explain that this important position would require extensive travel and asked me to help cover his busy practice during his absences. Of course I agreed. As President of ASCO, Glick had many accomplishments: hiring the first CEO of the society, establishing the Cancer Policy and Clinical Affairs Department, expanding ASCO's efforts in

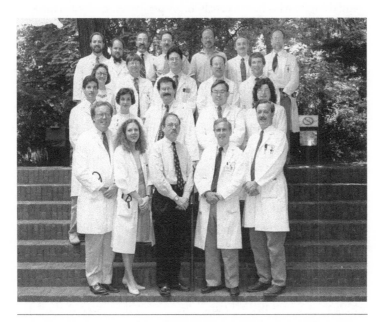

Figure 3. Division, 1993. Interim Division Chiefs Joel Bennett and John Glick are in the front row, third and fourth from left, respectively.

development of clinical practice guidelines, initiating the joint ASCO/AACR clinical trial methodology course for medical oncology fellows, and furthering ASCO's close relationship with the National Coalition for Cancer Survivorship. Fittingly, the 1996 ASCO meeting was held in Philadelphia. As Glick presided over this meeting, listening to his presidential address and attending the president's reception in the Philadelphia Museum of Art, I felt a tremendous sense of pride that my mentor was president of this great organization.

_____

While Glick and Bennett served as interim Division Co-Chiefs, the search for our next leader was on. Holmes invited Stephen Emerson to interview for the job. Emerson was a Harvard-trained hematologist who had recently been promoted to Associate Professor of Medicine at the University of Michigan. In his laboratory, he studied bone marrow stem-cell biology, especially as it related to bone marrow transplantation. He was young, enthusiastic, and highly intelligent. When I met with him for the first time, he nonchalantly asked me, "So how are you going to cure cancer?" In 1994, Emerson accepted Holmes's offer and became the third Chief of the Division of Hematology/Oncology, a position he held until 2007.

When Emerson arrived, he identified several deficiencies in our Division and strategically set out to fill them. The Division was very limited in fundamental research in cancer biology. Emerson recalled, "My first recruit was Wafik El-Deiry, a cancer biologist, the first one recruited here since Mark Greene and Peter Nowell. We didn't have one in the Department of Medicine."[2] El-Deiry received his MD and PhD in biochemistry at the University of Miami School of Medicine. He then completed his internal medicine and medical oncology training at Johns Hopkins. As a fellow he worked in the laboratory of Bert Vogelstein. There he discovered p21, or WAF1 (aptly named for himself), the first mammalian cell cycle inhibitor ever discovered. His paper, published in *Cell*, is one of the most-cited cancer biology papers of all time.[3] El-Deiry spent ten years in the Division and rose through the ranks to become Professor of Medicine, Genetics, and Pharmacology. In addition to continuing his groundbreaking research on p21, he discovered the TRAIL death receptor 5 (DR5) and defined the role of the extrinsic cell death pathway through p53 regulation of DR5.[4] In 2010, he was recruited to Penn State University to be Chief of Hematology/Oncology. Currently, he is Director of the Cancer Center at Brown University.

Emerson was concerned that the Division did not perform allogeneic bone marrow/stem cell transplants. It had a robust autologous bone marrow transplant program led by Edward Stadtmauer. However, Emerson saw allogeneic transplantation as the future of transplantation, especially for such diseases as acute leukemia. With allogeneic transplantation, bone marrow was harvested from a donor. After the patient received chemotherapy, the donor's allogeneic cells were infused or transplanted into the patient. The allogeneic stem cells resulted in a graft versus leukemia immunologic effect. At the time, most major centers, such as Memorial Sloan Kettering and Johns Hopkins, were performing allogeneic transplants. In fact, if we had a patient who required an allogeneic transplant, we would often refer them to these other centers.

Emerson was very interested in recruiting David Porter, who at the time was a second-year instructor at the Brigham and Women's Hospital doing allogeneic transplantation. The hospital had one of the largest bone marrow transplant programs in the country. During his hematology fellowship at Brigham and Women's,

Porter performed a very innovative pilot study in which he infused allogeneic donor T cells into patients with refractory chronic myelogenous leukemia and demonstrated that patients could experience durable remissions through a graft versus leukemia effect. Porter published these results in the *New England Journal of Medicine* when he was a third-year fellow.[5]

Emerson met with Porter at a bone marrow transplantation conference in Keystone, Colorado, and invited him to visit Penn. One day in 1999, Emerson called me into his office and told me he needed my help with something very important. "I really want Porter to come to Penn. I need you and Annie to take him out to dinner and show him that Penn is a great place to be at and that people here are normal." In fact, Annie and Porter already knew each other, having been medical school classmates at Brown. We happily agreed (if nothing else, it meant a great dinner billed to the Division). We took Porter to a famous Philadelphia Italian restaurant called the Saloon and had a great evening. Porter ultimately decided to join our Division to became Director of Allogeneic Bone Marrow Transplantation.

I asked Porter to reflect on how he was able to come to a new institution as a young faculty member and set up an allogeneic bone marrow transplantation program. "A lot of support from people at the Brigham. It seemed nuts that two years out of fellowship, someone was going to give me this opportunity. I didn't think something like this came along often. I had about a six-month lead time. I learned everything I could. I brought protocols and consent forms with me. We didn't have a lot of SOPs [standard operating procedures] back in the day. I brought all the protocols. I brought our procedures, our policies. I brought consent forms for various trials. I had lots of structure. I knew how things worked in the Brigham."[6]

Allogeneic bone marrow transplantation can be accompanied by life-threatening toxicity. Porter remembered that the initial patients treated at Penn did poorly. "I remember at one point that nine of our first ten patients ended up dying. Some died of toxicity. Some of them got through fine and relapsed. I was only three years out of fellowship and feeling tremendously insecure. What are we doing wrong? It was a hard time, but we pushed on." He was encouraged both by his former colleagues at Brigham and Women's and by Emerson to stay the course. Over the ensuing years, Porter built the Penn allogeneic transplantation program into one of the largest in the country.

During the 1990s, the hereditary basis of breast cancer was of great research interest. Several laboratories competed to identify the genes involved in hereditary breast cancer. In 1994, Emerson and Glick recruited Barbara Weber, a nationally recognized University of Michigan medical oncologist with expertise in the molecular genetics of hereditary breast cancer. Emerson knew Weber well since they had been colleagues at Michigan. At Penn, Weber established a laboratory research program in hereditary breast cancer. She played an important role in identifying *BRCA-2* as a hereditary breast cancer gene and was the first to demonstrate its importance in male breast cancer.[7] Perhaps even more important were the studies she led that have helped to set standards of care for patients with *BRCA-1/2*–related breast cancer. Weber and colleagues demonstrated that bilateral prophylactic mastectomy reduced the risk of breast cancer in women with these mutations by approximately 90 percent.[8] They also demonstrated that bilateral prophylactic oophorectomy substantially reduced the risk of breast cancer in women with the mutations.[9]

Weber mentored young investigators who would ultimately become highly respected researchers in hereditary cancer, including

the medical oncologist Susan Domchek, the molecular epidemiologist Timothy Rebbeck, and the medical geneticist Kate
Nathanson. Weber also established Penn's Cancer Risk Evaluation
Program, one of the first such programs in the country, to counsel
patients concerning their risk of hereditary cancer. She hired full-
time genetic counselors to support this endeavor. In 2005, Weber
left Penn for a position in the pharmaceutical industry. Her trainees,
including Domchek, carried on and rapidly built out hereditary
cancer research and care at Penn.

Emerson's recruitment of the developmental biologist Peter
Klein is a great example of his vision and creativity as a Division
Chief. Klein received his MD and PhD at Johns Hopkins and
then went to Massachusetts General Hospital, where he short-
tracked in internal medicine and completed his postdoctoral
work.[10] When he was recruited to Penn's Hematology/Oncology
faculty, Klein had not trained in either hematology or medical oncology. However, Emerson thought that Klein was too good a
scientist to pass up. Once on the faculty, Emerson constructed
for him a hematology fellowship track that included the opportunity to see patients in his clinic. Klein completed the fellowship requirements and became board-certified in hematology in
2008. Studying frog developmental biology, Klein was the first to
show that valproic acid functioned as a histone deacetylase inhibitor.[11] While seeing patients with myelodysplastic syndrome
(MDS) in Emerson's clinic, he had an idea: to use the chromatin-
modifying agent valproic acid in MDS. Emerson brought Klein
together with Selina Luger and the hematopathologist Adam
Bagg, and within six months they were treating MDS patients
with valproic acid in an approved investigator-initiated clinical
trial.

When I joined the faculty in 1993, the Division did not have a strong developmental therapeutics focus. Lynn Schuchter was doing innovative investigator-initiated clinical trials in melanoma, but most of the clinical trials were large studies conducted through the NCI Cooperative Group Program. In fact, we rarely had phase I trials of novel drugs available to our patients with refractory cancer. We would often send these patients across town to either Fox Chase Cancer Center or Thomas Jefferson University. Peter O'Dwyer had led developmental therapeutics programs at both institutions and was well recognized in the field and well connected with the pharmaceutical industry. In 1998, Emerson and Glick recruited O'Dwyer and his junior associate James Stevenson to establish Penn's Developmental Therapeutics Group. Initially, O'Dwyer and his group treated patients in a newly developed Clinical Investigations Unit at Presbyterian Hospital. With their arrival, we now had a robust portfolio of early-phase clinical trials that we could offer our patients with refractory cancer. The contributions of O'Dwyer and colleagues will be discussed later when we visit the era of targeted therapy because of the important role that they played not only at Penn but nationally.

In the 1990s at Penn, "gene therapy" was a major institutional effort. Kelley recruited James Wilson to establish and lead the Institute for Human Gene Therapy, the first of its kind in the country. At the Cancer Center, the Gene Therapy in Cancer Program was established by Glick in 1993. This program was led by Stephen Eck, who was recruited to our Division from the University of Michigan by Emerson, Glick, and Wilson. Eck led the development of several cancer gene therapy trials during his years at Penn, including a pilot trial of intratumoral injection of an adenovirus that expresses CD80 (B7-1) in melanoma (in collaboration with

Schuchter) and a phase I study of an adenovirus-expressing herpes simplex virus thymidine kinase in refractory brain tumors (in collaboration with Jane Alavi).

During his years as Division chief, Emerson emphasized expansion of the Hematologic Malignancies and Bone Marrow Transplantation groups. Luger, my co-fellow, joined the Division to focus on leukemia and novel drug development. Collaborating with Alan Gewirtz, she performed the first pilot trial of *c-myb* anti-sense therapy for refractory chronic myelogenous leukemia. For many years Luger served the Division as Director of the Leukemia Program until she stepped down in 2019. Keith Pratz was subsequently recruited from Johns Hopkins to assume leadership in leukemia. Martin Carroll, who trained at Harvard, was recruited to build a translational laboratory program in leukemia. While working with Emerson to build a human hematopoietic stem cell bank, he concurrently collected leukemia specimens. His acute myeloid leukemia (AML) tissue core has approximately 3,200 collections over a twenty-year period. This is one of the largest collections of viably frozen leukemia samples in the world.[12]

Glick was the most well-known lymphoma specialist not only in the Division but in Philadelphia. However, he could not possibly see all the patients with lymphoma who presented to Penn. Initially, he referred many to Kevin Fox and me, but he recognized the need for building a team whose primary focus would be lymphoma. He and Emerson recruited Stephen Schuster from Jefferson to lead our lymphoma group. Schuster shared with me the first phone call from Glick he received about coming to Penn. "I was in my lab on a Friday night and the internal line phone rings. 'Steve? This is John Glick.' and I'm like, 'Wow.' We had shared a couple of patients, and recently I had sent him a patient whom he sent back to me, so I assumed he was calling me to talk about the patient. And he goes, 'Steve, you know I was thinking about it, and we need someone like you at Penn. I think you would fit in with the Hematologic Malignancy group. I want to focus more on breast cancer, and I'd like to do less lymphoma.'"[13] Schuster came to Penn in 1998 and became the Director of Lymphoma, a position he holds to this day. His career at Penn has been highlighted by his recent successful use of CAR-T cell therapy in refractory lymphomas.

On the solid tumor side of the Division, the expansion of faculty was more modest. Joseph Treat was recruited to the Division as a lung cancer medical oncologist and clinical trialist. In academic medicine, there was an accepted truth that moving from private practice to an academic institution was not a likely career trajectory. As he usually did, Emerson continued to think outside the box. Kenneth Algazy led a private practice group in the Frankford area of Philadelphia but was looking for a change. He was recruited to Penn to focus on head and neck cancer but was a generalist as well. Algazy served as Chief of Hematology/Oncology at the Veterans Hospital until he retired from Penn in 2016.

An important factor in the Philadelphia health care market in the 1990s was the expansion of Allegheny Health Education and Research Foundation (AHERF). AHERF was established in 1983 with Allegheny General Hospital, a 670-bed hospital in Pittsburgh that was a teaching affiliate of the University of Pittsburgh.[14] In 1986, Sherif Abdelhak became CEO of this system with the goal of broadening its reach across the state of Pennsylvania. AHERF rapidly expanded into both the Pittsburgh and the Philadelphia markets by acquiring several hospitals, two medical schools (Medical College of Pennsylvania and Hahnemann Medical College), and many primary care and subspecialty physicians. Abdelhak recruited faculty from many local institutions, including Penn. In fact, one prominent otorhinolaryngologist was recruited away from Penn with the promise of having busy surgical practices in both Pittsburgh and Philadelphia and the use of a private jet to shuttle him back and forth.

AHERF approached faculty in the Division of Hematology/ Oncology at Penn with the promise of much higher salaries. Glick, a master of faculty retention, called me one day and said, "David, you may be getting a call from Allegheny asking you to come interview for a job at a much higher salary. This is not what it may seem to be." Emerson recognized that indeed the call of AHERF was not the promise of more opportunities but more money. He recognized that our salaries were inadequate and sought to change this. He proposed to the hospital administration that a proportion of the chemotherapy revenues be returned to the Division so that he could increase salaries. In conjunction with the Department of Medicine he also initiated a clinical productivity incentive plan. Because of Emerson's efforts, faculty salaries substantially increased. It is much to the credit of Glick and Emerson that the Division remained almost whole during these turbulent times: only one of our clinical faculty moved to AHERF; the rest remained at Penn. It was a good thing; in July 1998 AHERF filed for a $1.3 billion bankruptcy, the largest nonprofit health care failure in our country's history.

The late 1990s were tumultuous times for UPHS. In December 1995 the Office of the Inspector General announced that the Clinical Practices of the University of Pennsylvania (CPUP) would pay a $30 million fine to Medicare. Because of the changing reimbursement environment in Philadelphia, as well as the reductions in Medicare payments because of the Balanced Budget

Act, the previously financially sound health system began to experience losses: in 1998 to 2001 the health system lost $400 million. In addition, the death of a patient enrolled in one of the gene therapy trials in September 1999 led to the FDA halting gene therapy trials at Penn.

To curb financial losses, the health system hired the Hunter Group as a consultant. This group was known for a "slash-and-burn" approach to reform, and their ultimate recommendation was to cut all health system staff by 20 percent across the board. This alarmed many in the faculty, who already felt like they were practicing medicine on a shoestring budget. In December 2000, a rumor emerged that the university was considering sale of its health system to the for-profit group Vanguard Health Systems of Nashville. Under the leadership of Glick and others, the faculty of the medical school met and unanimously protested any potential sale of the health system. The university knew that it had to rethink its options. In November 2001, Penn announced the creation of "Penn Medicine," which included the medical school, CPUP, and the hospitals. Penn Medicine would be overseen by a new board, separate from the university's. By 2002, the health system was no longer losing money, and the financial turnaround had begun. I remember these tumultuous times well. I remember being interviewed by someone from the Hunter Group. I remember attending the faculty meeting protesting the sale of the health system. But I also remember feeling like life in our Division was stable and that Glick and Emerson were watching our backs throughout this turbulent time.

In 1998, the Hematology/Oncology outpatient practices moved from the sixth floor of Penn Tower to occupy the fourteenth and sixteenth floors. The fourteenth floor was eventually dedicated to the Rena Rowan Breast Center, the history of which will be discussed later. On this floor, a patient with breast cancer could experience true multidisciplinary care with simultaneous visits with surgery, medical oncology, and radiation oncology. This approach would set the standard at Penn for what would be coming later across the Cancer Center. The remainder of Hematology/Oncology patients were seen on the sixteenth floor and eventually the fifteenth floor. Despite this increase in space, we rapidly outgrew it, resulting in room shortages and prolonged waiting times for patients. It was not uncommon to see patients sitting on the window ledge waiting to be called. In addition, patients would often wait for hours for an infusion chair so that they could receive chemotherapy. We clearly needed a new outpatient center.

Pennsylvania Hospital, the nation's first hospital, was founded in 1751 by Benjamin Franklin and Thomas Bond. This hospital had long had an affiliation with the medical school, and many providers had adjunct faculty appointments. Pennsylvania Hospital was a favorite place for Penn medical students to do their rotations to get a taste of "real-world" medicine. Due to financial woes in the 1990s, Pennsylvania Hospital had to merge with a larger entity. Although Jefferson courted Pennsylvania Hospital, in 1996, it became part of the UPHS. However, physician practices were largely private practices. Arthur "Chip" Staddon and David Henry trained in Penn's Internal Medicine and Hematology/Oncology training programs. After establishing a private practice at the Graduate Hospital, this group moved to Pennsylvania Hospital when Graduate Hospital closed. They built a superb private practice in hematology and oncology. A unique aspect of this group is that although all members practiced general hematology/oncology, some established national reputations as oncology subspecialists. Staddon was a well-recognized sarcoma specialist. Henry was a national expert for AIDS-related malignancies.[15] This practice grew in stature and eventually became one of the largest private practice groups in the region and in fact competed for patients with our own Hematology/Oncology Division. However, the relationship between these private practice physicians and Penn faculty was always cordial.

Presbyterian Hospital was founded in 1871 and for many years was an independent community hospital affiliated with Penn but with its own board of directors. In 1995, Penn bought Presbyterian Hospital, renaming it the Presbyterian Medical Center of the University of Pennsylvania. Since Presbyterian was now owned by Penn, Emerson was responsible for building Hematology/Oncology there. He recruited Jack Goldberg to serve as Chief of Hematology/Oncology at Presbyterian. Goldberg was well known in the Philadelphia area for his expertise in benign hematology and hematologic malignancies. Goldberg subsequently recruited Gamil Hanna to assist him. Presbyterian also had a treatment center in Cherry Hill, New Jersey, which was staffed by Goldberg and Hanna.

In 1996, UPHS opened an outpatient facility in Radnor, Pennsylvania, a suburb of Philadelphia. When it was envisioned, Kelley planned that this facility would be staffed by full-time faculty from Penn. At that time, several faculty including Haller would spend one half-day per week at that facility. Over time, the health system recognized that this approach was not efficient or effective. Eventually, Staddon and Henry decided that their private practice would also practice in the Radnor facility.

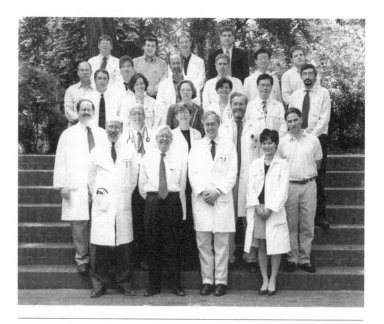

Figure 4. Division, 2000. Division Chief Stephen Emerson is in the front row, third from left.

In retrospect, the 1990s were important years for the Division. Emerson recruited strategically, giving the Division much more breadth, both scientifically and clinically. The Division remained whole during these troubled times. And then came a transformational gift that changed the course of history for both the Division and the Cancer Center.

EIGHT

The Transformational Gift

A s I interviewed members of our faculty, I asked what they saw as seminal events in the evolution of the Division. Many felt that a major change occurred with the establishment of the Abramson Family Cancer Research Institute (AFCRI) in 1999. As background, Madlyn Abramson, a graduate of the University of Pennsylvania, was a breast cancer survivor who was treated by John Glick. Her husband, Leonard Abramson, is credited with the development of health maintenance organizations, or HMOs, in the 1980s. He founded U.S. Healthcare Inc., one of the country's first HMOs. In 1996, he sold U.S. Healthcare to Aetna.

In his role as Cancer Center Director, Glick approached the Abramsons about making a major gift to Penn that would transform cancer care. For two years, Glick and the Abramsons negotiated the specifics of this gift. In 1997, the Abramsons made a $100 million commitment to Penn to establish the AFCRI. This is especially remarkable considering the financial troubles that the health system was experiencing at the time. Mr. Abramson was on the Board of Trustees at Johns Hopkins University and strongly considered giving the gift to Johns Hopkins. But Mrs. Abramson was loyal to her alma mater and especially to Glick, her oncologist. In the end, Penn was the fortunate recipient of this remarkable gift. The vision that the Abramsons and Glick had was that the AFCRI would recruit world-class researchers to Penn "to propel cancer research to an exceptional level and to foster the development of innovative translational research."[1] Further, the Abramsons emphasized that in addition to cancer care at Penn being the best available anywhere, it should also be highly personalized and comprehensive, not just for those with means but for all patients. In recognition of the extraordinary support and vision of the Abramsons, Glick persuaded Penn president Judith Rodin to rename the Cancer Center as the Abramson Cancer Center (ACC) of the University of Pennsylvania in June 2002.

The AFCRI rapidly became an integral component of the Cancer Center. When the AFCRI was established, Glick, who was then the Director of the Cancer Center, was named President of this new organization. His first step was to recruit a Scientific Director of the institute. Stephen Emerson suggested to the search committee a colleague from his days at Michigan, Craig Thompson. After a national search, Glick recruited Thompson in 1999 to be the AFCRI's first Scientific Director. Thompson graduated from the University of Pennsylvania School of Medicine in 1977. After completing fellowship training in medical oncology at the Fred Hutchinson Cancer Research Center, he was recruited in 1987 to the University of Michigan by William Kelley, then Michigan's Chair of Medicine. Thompson relocated to the University of Chicago in 1993, where he remained until he was recruited to Penn. As Kelley told me, "As far as I was concerned, Craig was the right guy for the job."[2] Michael Parmacek, Penn's current Chair of Medicine, recalled, "When Craig came, I think that there was a fundamental change in the place in terms of cancer biology. Craig is one of the most creative scientists I've ever met in my life. He's like a fountain of ideas, some of which are just crazy, but his crazy ideas turn into major discoveries. His personality lights up a room, he is charismatic, he is not shy, and he tells you what he is thinking. When you're building a program, it can be very catalytic to have somebody like Craig. With the resources that the Abramsons provided, he recruited excellent faculty. From a scientific standpoint, he expanded Penn's excellence beyond platelet biology in terms of basic and translational science into new directions."[3]

As Scientific Director, Thompson, in collaboration with Glick, recruited several world-class investigators to Penn and placed Penn on the map as a leader in fundamental and translational cancer research. These included Celeste Simon, a molecular biologist who studied cancer cell metabolism, tumor immunology, and cellular responses to oxygen deprivation; Gary Koretzky, a rheumatologist who studied T cell receptor signaling; Lewis Chodosh, an endocrinologist with a laboratory focused on cancer biology and in particular breast cancer; and Carl June, an immunologist and translational researcher who focused on the development of novel T cell therapies to treat cancer and HIV. Importantly, these investigators were recruited from outside of Penn to bring their unique expertise to the institution. It is noteworthy that these investigators came from a variety of disciplines, not only hematology/oncology. These researchers and many others who have been recruited to the AFCRI have transformed Penn into a world-renowned center for fundamental and translational research in cancer biology.

The impact of the AFCRI has been far-reaching and profound. From 1998 to 2018, NCI funding at Penn increased from $23.8 million to $72.7 million; the number of full-time Hematology/ Oncology faculty increased from 40 to 125; endowed professorships at the Cancer Center increased from 12 to 53; and Cancer Center philanthropy increased from $2.8 million to $38 million annually. Without the support of the AFCRI, it is doubtful that the eventual successful development of CAR-T therapy would have happened. By any measure, the Abramson gift has been transformational for the Division and the ACC. Because of their gift, both adults and children with refractory types of cancer who otherwise would have died are being cured with CAR-T therapy. Parmacek summed up the impact of the Abramson gift best: "Few people have given gifts that have not only transformed the institution but the whole field of cancer research."

NINE

The New Millennium

A s the new millennium started, the Division and the ACC were continuing to grow. In November 2000, the ACC opened the Rena Rowan Breast Center. John Glick recalled for me how this center came to be. "In the late 1990s, it became apparent that we were desperately short of ambulatory space in Penn Tower. We simply did not have enough infusion or exam rooms, and our patients were waiting for hours to see a physician or to receive their chemotherapy. We knew that the Health System was having financial difficulties and could not afford to fund any additional space. At that time, we visited the Evelyn Lauder Breast Center at Memorial Sloan Kettering in New York City. This center served as a model for what we wanted to do at Penn. I made an appointment with Dean Kelley and proposed the idea of a Breast Center at Penn. He said he could not fund it. I then proposed that we would raise the money from grateful patients to design, construct, and furnish the Breast Center so it would be a turnkey operation with no cost to the Health System. A vacant floor on Penn Tower would be the site of the new center. Dean Kelley smiled and said that if I could raise the money, we could build the center. Four months later I returned to his office with $4 million in signed gift commitments, including $1 million from Rena Rowan to name the center and $1 million from Sidney Kimmel. Dean Kelley was somewhat flabbergasted but said okay, you did it, and you have permission to go ahead with the full project. The Rena Rowan Breast Center would include multiple exam and consultation rooms, dedicated physician offices for the breast medical oncologists, and an infusion area for patients with breast cancer. In addition to medical oncology, radiation oncologists and breast cancer surgeons would see patients in the new center, as did the lymphedema specialists and psychosocial counselors. The center also included a boutique for our patients. Rena herself helped design the fabrics and furnishings. All of this was accomplished in two years from the first proposal in 1998 to the opening of the center in November 2020. Later, when the Perelman Center for Advanced Medicine was being constructed, Rena Rowan and her husband, Vic Damone, gave another $2 million to move and name the Rena Rowan Breast Center on the third floor of Perelman. Their kindness and generosity will always be remembered."[1]

When the Rowan Breast Center opened, Kevin Fox was named Medical Director. Fox, who was a key person in the development of the center, told me, "We decided we would create basically a multidisciplinary, physical space where people with breast cancer could come and get all elements of their care. A simple concept. Its long-term success was going to be measured only in three ways. One is that patients would have to show up and be happy about it, and they have. The second would be we could do this and be an asset financially, scientifically, and educationally to the institution, which we have. The third and the most elusive is the development of a sustained clinical research program within the Breast Center. The third was always going to be the biggest challenge of all. I think we're finally at a point where our now junior and senior faculty have established legitimate academic careers in clinical investigation."[2] Although many have contributed to the success of the breast cancer clinical research program, Fox gives much of the credit to his colleague Angela DeMichele.

Between her third and fourth years of medical school, DeMichele participated in a research program called the Four Schools Physician/Scientist Scholars Program, which allowed her to spend a year doing research in a laboratory at either Washington University, Penn, Johns Hopkins, or Duke University. She spent a year at Penn in the laboratory of Doug Cines, and her project was an analysis of the antiphospholipid antibody syndrome and its association with fetal loss. In 1994, she started her internship in obstetrics and gynecology at Penn, which consisted of six months of internal medicine and six months of obstetrics/gynecology. During her medicine block, she was an intern on the Silverstein 7 Oncology Unit and Fox was her attending. It was a transformational experience: she knew then that she wanted to switch into internal medicine and then train in hematology/oncology.

When DeMichele started her fellowship, there were only three women on the faculty (Lynn Schuchter, Jane Alavi, and Selina Luger; Janet Abrahm had left Penn for Harvard) and none had children. DeMichele became pregnant during her first year of fellowship and delivered her first son during the second year. Having a child during fellowship was highly unusual at the time.

DeMichele also earned a master's of science in clinical epidemiology during her second and third years of training. This, too, was unusual, although now many of our fellows earn a master's degree as part of their research experience. For her research, she worked with Barbara Weber on breast cancer genetics. She learned breast cancer clinical medicine in Fox's clinic.

In 2000, DeMichele joined the Division as a breast cancer oncologist. At the time there was little clinical research ongoing. The Division attempted to recruit a well-known breast cancer clinical trialist but failed. "I remember Kevin calling me into his office and saying, 'I'm going to recommend that they just hire you for this job, and you'll be the person to try to build clinical trials and clinical research here,' which was great. I felt so supported. There was maybe one ECOG trial, but that was when Herceptin was in clinical trials. I remember thinking, 'We need to open trials with Herceptin; this looks interesting and important.' The first trials I opened were Herceptin trials. That was sort of my introduction because the era of targeted therapy was happening. It was an exciting time to try to be doing clinical trials because there were all these new drugs. We started opening trials and using these drugs."[3] She has continued conducting very important translational research in breast cancer, leads the Breast Cancer Program of the ACC, and is the first chair holder of the Jill and Alan Miller Professorship in Breast Cancer Excellence.

DeMichele sees Schuchter as an outstanding mentor and role model for her, as well as a very close friend. "It's hard to put into words even the enormity of her influence because it's on so many levels. We were pregnant at the same time, her twins, my second son. I was going through this with someone." Reflecting on mentorship, she said, "If you really want to know why do I do breast cancer? Kevin Fox. Why do I have an academic career and do clinical trials and research? Lynn Schuchter. They have really been the people who've been incredible to me."

In 2001, Craig Thompson, John Glick, and Stephen Emerson recruited Robert Vonderheide to Penn. Vonderheide, a Rhodes scholar who trained in medicine and medical oncology at Harvard, was on the faculty at the Dana Farber Cancer Institute where his focus was immunotherapy. His wife, Susan Domchek, who was completing her fellowship at the Farber was simultaneously recruited for the breast cancer program. Vonderheide recalled their recruitment. "When Susan and I left Penn after that first visit, we looked at each other and said, 'We're coming to Penn.' It was obvious. It's an interesting question to think back to why we were so sure. When we came to Penn and started talking to leaders, it was all about growth. The Abramson Family Cancer Research Institute was relatively new. It had only been going for three years, but it was recruiting major investigators in many departments from all over the country."[4] He recalls discussing this with senior leadership at the Farber who felt like they were making a big mistake, citing the gene therapy incident and the financial situation. "Our reaction was, 'It's the University of Pennsylvania. It's the oldest medical school in the country. It has a storied history. It's going to gain momentum. It's only going up. We wanted to be a part of helping to build it.'" As we will see later, Vonderheide's impact at Penn has been extraordinary.

Domchek worked with Judy Garber, a breast cancer geneticist, during her medical oncology fellowship at the Dana Farber Cancer Institute. She recalled, "I graduated from medical school in 1995, so I grew up with the search for *BRCA1/2*. Back at that time no one knew what these genes did or what were the risks associated with these genes. Barb [Weber] had a lead role in figuring this out. When I came here, Barb was doing some of the clinical work but was more interested in the lab. She said, 'You do the clinical side.'"[5] Domchek took a lead role in the Cancer Risk Evaluation Program. When Weber left Penn in 2005, Domchek became the leader of the Breast Cancer Genetics Program.

———

The Division continued to grow under Emerson with key recruitments in hematologic malignancy, solid tumor, and benign hematology. Alison Loren joined the faculty in 2003. Her main interests were leukemia and bone marrow transplantation. While she was a fellow, David Porter was her primary mentor, and she credits him with her career direction. When DuPont Guerry retired in 2009, Loren, who had served as his Associate Director of the fellowship program, became the Director. In this position, she took great personal interest in each of our fellows and met with them regularly to provide career guidance. Reflecting on this experience, she states, "It was really, for me, honoring DuPont's legacy of keeping this place as a true academic, intellectual environment that cares about the right things."[6] She served as Fellowship Director through 2016, when she accepted a position as Vice Chair of Medicine for Faculty Development. She was recently named Director of Blood and Marrow Transplantation for the Division.

Sunita Nasta, who trained in lymphoma at the M. D. Anderson Cancer Center, was brought on in 2001 to work with Schuster. Nasta continues at Penn and leads the much-beloved Thursday-morning fellows' tumor board. Donald Tsai who trained in our fellowship joined the faculty in 2000. Tsai has become one of the leading authorities on post-transplant lymphoproliferative disease.

Alexander "Sasha" Perl was recruited from Johns Hopkins to do translational research in AML. Perl's research focuses on molecularly targeted therapeutics for acute leukemia. One of his areas of expertise is in FLT3 inhibitors for AML, and he has played a leading role in clinical trials of these agents. Elizabeth Hexner worked closely with Scott Murphy when she was a fellow. Murphy was a member of the original Polycythemia Vera Study Group, a historic effort that resulted in better understanding of how to best manage myeloproliferative disorders. Following in his footsteps, Hexner created the Penn Center for Myeloproliferative Neoplasms.

On the solid tumor side, there also was growth, especially in gastrointestinal (GI) oncology. Weijing Sun was recruited out of our fellowship to help Haller with the GI oncology program (which needed help since I was now focused on GU cancer). Sun had an interest in upper GI tract and hepatobiliary cancer. After serving on our faculty, he later joined the University of Pittsburgh and in 2017 was named Director of the Medical Oncology Division at the University of Kansas. In 2005, Ursina Teitelbaum was recruited to Penn to focus on GI oncology. She had trained at the University of Chicago and was board certified not only in medical oncology but also in geriatrics. Teitelbaum is recognized for her outstanding clinical care and is a member of Penn Medicine's Academy of Master Clinicians. Bruce Giantonio was recruited from Fox Chase Cancer Center to practice GI oncology. Giantonio also was Executive Officer of ECOG-ACRIN. He served as the principal investigator on E3200, a randomized trial of 5-FU, leucovorin, and oxaliplatin (FOLFOX4) with or without bevacizumab in the second-line treatment of patients with metastatic colorectal cancer, that demonstrated a survival benefit with the addition of bevacizumab.[7] Giantonio left Penn in 2016 to join the faculty at Massachusetts General Hospital and is greatly missed.

Tracey Evans was a graduate of Penn's Medical School. After training in medicine and medical oncology at Harvard where she worked with Thomas Lynch at Massachusetts General, she joined our faculty to focus on thoracic oncology. Evans also played a major role in quality-improvement programs for the Division until she left to join the staff at Lankenau Medical Center. Naomi Haas was recruited from Fox Chase Cancer Center. Haas has expertise in prostate cancer and renal cancer, which balanced nicely with my interests in testicular cancer and bladder cancer. She was accomplished in clinical trials and served in leadership positions in ECOG-ACRIN.

The benign hematology program also experienced growth. The Children's Hospital of Philadelphia sits adjacent to the Hospital of the University of Pennsylvania. The Division of Hematology at CHOP is well recognized for excellence in patient care and basic and translational research. CHOP has very strong programs in hemophilia, sickle cell disease, and thalassemia. These programs were noticeably absent in our Division. This was problematic, especially for those pediatric patients who were aging out of CHOP and needed an adult hematologist. Emerson recognized the importance of building these programs, especially in hemophilia. In 2000, he recruited Barbara Konkle from Jefferson to establish and lead the Penn Comprehensive Hemophilia and Thrombosis Program. Konkle was well known for her expertise and research in hemophilia and von Willebrand's disease. Konkle focused not only on building the clinical program but also on developing its research and education arms. She was the principal investigator of a K–12 training grant for mentored career development in clinical research in nonmalignant hematology, providing support for fellows interested in an academic career in that area. In 2009, Konkle was recruited to the University of Washington and Bloodworks Northwest in Seattle.

———

The Developmental Therapeutics Group was extraordinarily productive in the development of targeted therapies for cancer. During the research year of his fellowship, Keith Flaherty worked with Peter O'Dwyer to build this program, and he joined the Division in 2002. These early investigational trials were initially performed at Presbyterian Medical Center's Clinical Investigations Unit. In 2008, the Developmental Therapeutics group moved to the Perelman Center for Advanced Medicine, and in 2016 a dedicated phase I unit opened there. The importance of having a robust Developmental Therapeutics program at a comprehensive cancer center cannot be overstated. This is where firsts in human clinical trials of new agents are performed. In phase I trials, the investigators determine what is the safest and potentially most effective dose of a new agent to take into further testing. For our patients with metastatic disease who are out of treatment options but not ready for hospice care, phase I trials offer the opportunity for ongoing treatment, hopefully with an agent that biologically makes sense for the patient and that is beneficial and effective. In addition, when the Developmental Therapeutics group gains access to a new agent, other Division faculty have the chance to study the agent, perhaps helping to bring it into larger, disease-specific phase 2 trials.

The era of targeted therapy started in the late 1990s and continues today. Targeted therapy for cancer is based on inhibiting the growth of cancer cells by interfering with specific molecular targets that are needed for tumor growth. Targeted therapy emerged as our understanding of cancer genomics expanded. Imatinib is an example of a highly successful targeted approach for chronic myelogenous leukemia. The fusion protein BCR-ABL is critical for the development of CML; imatinib is a BCR-ABL tyrosine kinase inhibitor. In breast cancer, the drug trastuzamab, which is a monoclonal antibody that targets HER-2 neu, is an important treatment option for patients with HER-2-positive cancer. Of note, targeted therapy has the potential of being most effective when the cancer is less genetically complex. When a cancer has multiple mutations resulting in several active pathways driving its growth, targeted therapy becomes more challenging and combinations may be needed.

O'Dwyer and Flaherty led several important clinical trials in the early targeted therapy era. Flaherty was the principal investigator of a phase I/II trial of BAY 43-9006 in melanoma and renal cell cancer. This agent, later called sorafenib, gained FDA approval for the treatment of renal cell cancer.[8] Although it had modest single-agent activity in melanoma, Flaherty performed a phase I/II trial combining sorafenib with paclitaxel/carboplatin in melanoma, which led to an ECOG phase III trial chaired by Flaherty comparing paclitaxel and carboplatin with paclitaxel, carboplatin, and sorafenib. Although the addition of sorafenib to chemotherapy did not improve the outcome compared to chemotherapy alone, the trial was important in that it was one of the first to test the addition of a targeted agent to cytotoxic chemotherapy.[9]

Subsequent work focused on developing therapy for melanoma targeting the proto-oncogene *BRAF*. In the early 2000s, tumor biology investigators, including Helen Davies and Weber at Penn, found that activating mutations in *BRAF* were commonly seen in melanoma.[10] Flaherty led the first phase I trial of vemurafenib (then called PLX4032) in *BRAF* mutant metastatic melanoma. A large proportion of these patients benefited from this treatment.[11]

Penn accrued the largest number of patients with melanoma to this trial. It was followed by a large, international phase 3 trial that compared vemurafenib with the chemotherapy drug dacarbazine and demonstrated improved survival in patients treated with vemurafenib, ultimately leading to FDA approval.[12] Through the work of the Developmental Therapeutics Program and the Melanoma Program, Penn played a major role in the development of vemurafenib. Flaherty left Penn in 2008 to become Director of Experimental Therapeutics at the Massachusetts General Hospital Cancer Center. While a detailed description of subsequent melanoma trials is beyond the scope of this text, additional studies of BRAF inhibitors and MEK inhibitors, alone and in combination have resulted in significant advances for patients with melanoma. Schuchter and her junior colleagues Leslie Fescher (who subsequently left Penn to lead the melanoma program at Indiana University) and Tara Mitchell played significant roles in these trials.

Ravi Amaravadi trained as a fellow at Penn in Hematology/Oncology. He spent two years in Craig Thompson's laboratory studying a process called autophagy in cancer cells. Autophagy ("self-eating") is a process in which cells degrade intracellular proteins and organelles in lysosomes in order to recycle intracellular components to sustain metabolism and survival. Autophagy plays an important role in both normal and diseased states, including cancer. Amaravadi, a key member of the Developmental Therapeutics Group, has led several clinical trials targeting autophagy as treatment for cancer. Interestingly, the antimalarial drug hydroxychloroquine is an autophagy inhibitor, and he has combined this agent with several other anticancer drugs in a variety of cancer types.[13] Subsequently, Amaravadi, Thomas Karasic, and colleagues reported a randomized phase II trial of gemcitabine nab-paclitaxel with or without hydroxychloroquine in patients with advanced pancreatic cancer.[14] Presently, Amaravadi is leading the ECOG-ACRIN BAMM2 trial, which is a randomized, double-blind, phase II study of dabrafenib and trametinib with or without hydroxychloroquine in advanced *BRAF* V600E/K mutant melanoma. Amaravadi's work demonstrates the importance of having a robust Developmental Therapeutics program: innovative early-phase studies lead to larger disease-specific trials, which allow more patients to potentially benefit from this research.

———

In 2006, Glick decided to step down from his position as Cancer Center Director. He would continue to serve as President of the AFCRI and became Vice President for Resource Development for the health system and Associate Dean at the School of Medicine. Craig Thompson succeeded Glick as Director of the ACC. Arthur H. Rubenstein, who replaced Kelley as Executive Vice President of the University of Pennsylvania for the Health System and Dean of the School of Medicine, stated, "Dr. Thompson was selected for this position because of his reputation for excellence as a pioneer in cancer research, an exceptional educator, and above all, his career-long dedication to finding new approaches to treating and curing cancer."[15] Thompson served as Director of the ACC until 2010, when he left Penn to become President and CEO of Memorial Sloan Kettering Cancer Center in New York. When he stepped down as Scientific Director of the AFCRI, Celeste Simon was appointed to that position.

In 2007, Emerson called an urgent faculty meeting for an important announcement. We assembled in Agnew Grice Auditorium, which is a simulacrum of an anatomical theater. I remember sitting among my colleagues wondering what this was all about. Emerson walked and stood before us. "I want to let you know that I will be resigning as Division Chief. I am going to be the thirteenth

President of Haverford College, starting July 1, 2007. This is a dream come true because as many of you know I attended Haverford as an undergraduate and am a loyal alumnus." And thus, the Emerson as Division Chief era came to an end.

I think by any measure Emerson's tenure as Division Chief was highly successful. Some important metrics are worth considering. In 1993, the Division had 16 full-time faculty members, including 8 basic scientists and 8 clinicians. By 2006, the Division had 52 full-time faculty, 19 scientists on the tenure track, 24 clinician-educators, and 9 academic-clinicians. The outpatient visits grew from 11,000 per year to nearly 40,000. Chemotherapy infusions exceeded 22,000 per year. The inpatient bed census grew from 28 to 74. Research funding grew from $6 million to over $44 million annually, with 80 percent of this funding being derived from the NIH. Finally, Emerson expanded the fellowship from 4 fellows per year to 8 fellows per year. In addition, under his watch, the fellows were being recruited from the top internal medicine training programs nationally.[16] Emerson became the thirteenth President of Haverford in July 2007. He oversaw a faculty of 128 full- and part-time professors and a student body of 1,200 undergraduates.[17] He served as Haverford's President for four years. In February 2012, he became Director of the Herbert Irving Comprehensive Cancer Center at New York-Presbyterian Hospital/Columbia University Medical Center.

TEN

The Present Era

When Stephen Emerson resigned as Division Chief, the acting Chair of the Department of Medicine, Rick Shannon, asked Lynn Schuchter to serve as interim Division Chief. He then initiated a national search for Emerson's replacement. A series of external candidates and one internal candidate, Schuchter, were interviewed for this important position. Among the Hematology/Oncology faculty, there was only one choice for Division Chief and that was Schuchter. She was one of us, we knew her well, and we knew that her leadership would support all facets of this large, complex Division. In December 2008, Schuchter was named the fourth Chief of the Hematology/Oncology Division.

Shannon recalled, "When Steve Emerson decided to . . . become the president at Haverford, there was a really defining moment. I think the modern-day moment for the division. Historically, it had always been directed by a physician scientist, someone with a deep and compelling interest in basic research.

Yet, I saw this as an opportunity to really shift that phenotype from someone deeply rooted in basic science to someone who had a great clinical and translational research portfolio. Of course, that someone was Lynn Schuchter."[1] The present Chair of the Department of Medicine, Michael Parmacek, agreed: "Lynn was the perfect complement to really take the division to a new level. She had a very different leadership style than anybody that's been a division director before. She's obviously world-class—recognized for being a world-class clinician and doing outstanding clinical research, recognized internationally for the melanoma research that she's done. But that's not her most important strength. She has people skills and emotional intelligence and the ability to keep an all-star team together way beyond what most other people have."[2]

Throughout her career, Schuchter has been an outstanding role model for our faculty. In addition to her many academic achievements, Schuchter is the mother of twin sons who are college age. It is not surprising that women of the faculty look to her for career guidance as they attempt to achieve work-life balance. In 2017, she was the recipient of the FOCUS Award for the Advancement of Women in Medicine. This award recognizes a faculty member at Penn Medicine, male or female, whose outstanding efforts and achievements have promoted the career success, leadership, and overall quality of life for Penn women in academic medicine.

An important requirement for successfully leading the Hematology/Oncology Division is the ability to collaborate and work closely with the Director of the ACC. When Schuchter was named Division Chief, Craig Thompson was the fourth Director of the ACC. They established an excellent working relationship. Thompson, a member of the Hematology/Oncology Division, chose

Schuchter as his Associate Director for Clinical Research on the 2010 CCSG application, which received an "outstanding" rating by the NCI. They also worked closely as part of the Cancer Service Line to improve the delivery of cancer care at Penn. Schuchter told me, "I loved working with Craig. Craig would come to my office all the time to discuss different issues. It was a really good relationship between the Division and the Cancer Center. The boundaries were very clear. He was so great for the division; he brought in great people."[3]

When Thompson resigned in 2010 as Director of the ACC, Chi Van Dang was named the fifth Director of the ACC. John Glick chaired the search committee that recruited Dang from Johns Hopkins where he had served as Vice Dean for Research. He was trained as a medical oncologist and was very accomplished in fundamental cancer biology research. He was a complement to Schuchter with her focus on clinical and translational research. Dang was also a member of the Division of Hematology/Oncology. Of interest, all of the ACC Directors since Peter Nowell have been members of our Division. An especially innovative initiative under Dang was the development of Translational Centers of Excellence. These centers were funded through an internal grant mechanism and encouraged interdisciplinary and translational research. Three of them were initially awarded in breast cancer, lung cancer, and hematological malignancies. As ACC Director, Dang led the submission of the 2015 CCSG application, which was again considered "outstanding" by the NCI. In December 2016, he stepped down as ACC Director to become Scientific Director of the Ludwig Institute for Cancer Research.

Early in her tenure, Schuchter made several key recruitments to the Division. In 2010, she recruited Roger Cohen from Fox Chase Cancer Center. Cohen was Director of the Phase I program

at Fox Chase and was interim Division Chief of Hematology/
Oncology. He trained in internal medicine and hematology at
Mt. Sinai Hospital in New York. From 1989 through 1994, he
worked at the FDA, ultimately as Deputy Director of the Monoclonal Antibody Branch. He then became an oncologist with a
strong commitment to clinical trials. After being on the faculty at
the University of Virginia, he came to Fox Chase in 2001. He told
me, "I deliberately came to Philadelphia to work at the Fox Chase
Cancer Center because Fox Chase at that time was a clinical trials
powerhouse."[4] When he arrived at Fox Chase, he never would
have thought he would ultimately end up at Penn. However, Fox
Chase subsequently suffered administrative and financial strug-
gles that resulted in many of their faculty leaving. Cohen was
recruited to the Division not only as a thoracic and head-neck
oncologist and a phase I drug investigator but also to serve as
Associate Director for Clinical Research of the ACC. He put a
tremendous amount of effort into streamlining the clinical trial
process at Penn. One of his key initiatives was hiring a full-time
attorney for the Cancer Center who would focus on clinical trial
contracts. Under his guidance, the clinical trial activation process
at ACC greatly improved.

When Alison Loren stepped down as Director of our fellowship program in 2016, Schuchter asked Cohen to consider taking
this on. Cohen was regarded as a superb mentor for fellows and
junior faculty and was very committed to the academic mission of
the Division. He agreed to do this but only if there was a core of
junior faculty assisting him in the effort. Together, Cohen and his
assistant directors Erin Aarkus, Adam Cuker, and Kim Reiss-
Binder have done a superb job with the fellowship. I asked Cohen
about how he sees the state of the fellowship. "The fellowship is
strong, the fellowship is unique, the fellowship also benefits from

some resources that you have at Penn that you don't have other places. We have numerous training grants to support their second and third years of fellowship. Plus, we have all of these master's programs. Together these programs and training grants create synergies that you simply cannot realize in a place that doesn't have the resources that Penn has." Cohen was referring to the fact that Penn had master's programs in clinical epidemiology, translational research, and public policy that are available for many of the fellows during the second and third fellowship years. In 2021, Cohen stepped down and Aarkus was appointed fellowship director.

Schuchter was instrumental in recruiting Corey Langer from Fox Chase in 2008. Langer was an internationally known expert in lung cancer who was very active in clinical trials, both through the cooperative group mechanism and through industry. He was recruited to be Director of Thoracic Oncology with the charge of building this program. Cohen and Langer also recruited Charu Aggarwal to our faculty. Aggarwal trained with Cohen and Langer at Fox Chase and rapidly emerged at Penn as an outstanding thoracic oncologist. Schuchter also recruited Arati Desai from Johns Hopkins, where she trained with Stuart Grossman in neuro-oncology, and Nevena Damjanov from Temple. Damjanov was a Hematology/Oncology fellow at Penn, and she became Division chief at the Veterans Hospital when Kenneth Algazy stepped down.

⸺

For many years, Glick envisioned a free-standing ambulatory cancer building where all patients would experience the same sort of personalized care that our patients with breast cancer received at the Rena Rowan Breast Center. Through his determination and doggedness, Glick's dream became a reality. In the summer of

2008, the Perelman Center for Advanced Medicine (PCAM) opened its doors. The total cost for this project was $300 million, the largest amount ever committed by the Penn Health System. Ruth and Raymond Perelman generously gave $25 million for this building, and Glick raised an additional $25 million. PCAM was Glick's vision realized and enlarged. The spectacular building was designed by the renowned architect Rafael Viñoly and named in honor of Raymond and Ruth Perelman, whose philanthropy to the school of medicine and the health system was unsurpassed. At the dedication, Penn president Amy Gutman stated, "The Ruth and Raymond Perelman Center for Advanced Medicine exemplifies Penn's commitment to move from excellence to eminence in the care of patients and the creation of innovative treatments. This new facility is not only a fitting home for superb Penn doctors, scientists, nurses, and students who are the heart and soul of Penn Medicine, but also a powerful symbol of hope to patients and their families. It is a fitting tribute to the compassion and generosity of Ruth and Ray Perelman and their loyal and steadfast support for Penn." Arthur Rubenstein added, "In the life of a great academic medical center, there are certain defining moments that move it to the next level of excellence. For Penn Medicine, the Perelman Center for Advanced Medicine is one of those moments. This facility is a world-class center for the most exciting and promising clinical care, which will set a new standard for patient care."[5]

The west wing of this building was dedicated to the Abramson Cancer Center, with three outpatient oncology floors. Each floor consisted of many examination and consultation rooms, as well as individual chemotherapy infusion rooms. Each floor had its own laboratory facility for the coordination of laboratory testing, with dedicated space for research sample procurement and a dedicated pharmacy capable of preparing standard-of-care and investigational chemotherapeutic agents. The cancer-related outpatient activities of surgical, medical, and radiation oncology were coordinated within this combined facility. In addition, PCAM was designed to foster and accommodate the conduct of clinical trials and greatly facilitated the ACC's ability to effectively coordinate therapeutic and observational outpatient cancer research. More recently, the first floor of PCAM was converted to a patient care floor for benign hematology and cancer genetics.

The adjacent wings of PCAM house state-of-the-art cardiology, pulmonary, radiology, outpatient surgical operating rooms, and an endoscopy suite. Because many medical subspecialties occupy space contiguous to ours, there is easy and immediate access to subspecialty consultation for oncology patients. The Cardio-Oncology Program is a prime example. This unique center of excellence was founded by Penn cardiologist Joseph Carver, the Bernard Fishman Clinical Professor of Medicine at the Abramson Cancer Center of the University of Pennsylvania. The ACC's Patient and Family Services Programs were located on the first floor of PCAM. This center includes nutritional counseling, psychosocial counseling, patient navigation, a patient education center, and a boutique that specializes in cancer support products. In 2010, the Roberts Proton Therapy Center opened in PCAM, a first-of-its-kind facility that represented the only proton therapy available in the region. Glick raised $15 million from the Roberts family and helped secure Department of Defense funding for this project.

From a personal perspective, PCAM has made both being a patient and practicing oncology a much more enjoyable experience. From its open and light-filled design to increased patient capacity, the building has accomplished Glick's original goals and then some. Fittingly, on the first floor of the west pavilion, across from the elevators where patients are transported to their respective floor, hangs a portrait of Glick by world-renowned painter Nelson Shanks (1937–2015). It is a lasting tribute to the man who did the most to make PCAM a reality.

As evidenced by the Abramson and Perelman gifts, philanthropy can substantially alter the direction of an institution's development. The AFCRI established Penn as one of the world's leading centers for cancer biology basic research. PCAM transformed clinical care at Penn. Philanthropy has also played a major role in supporting the breast cancer program at Penn. Mariann MacDonald, who is a breast cancer survivor, and her husband, Robert, have been extraordinarily generous in their of support of the Division and the Cancer Center. Kevin Fox was named the first chair holder of the Mariann T. and Robert J. MacDonald Professorship in Breast Cancer Care Excellence. In addition, the MacDonalds' philanthropy resulted in the establishment of the Mariann and Robert MacDonald Cancer Risk Evaluation Center, which was founded in 2010. This center, located in the Rena Rowan Breast Center, focuses on genetic evaluation and medical management of individuals with inherited risk factors for cancer. When it was founded, Susan Domchek was named Director. Domchek told me, "We've been really fortunate over the years to have significant philanthropic support. . . . In 2010, there was the first large gift, which was from Mariann and Robert Macdonald, which provides funding for our genetic risk clinical program."[6]

In 2012, the Basser Center for BRCA at the Abramson Cancer Center was established. Mindy and Jon Gray, 1992 graduates of Penn, have given more than $70 million to support this center, named to honor Mindy's sister Faith Basser, who died of *BRCA*-related ovarian cancer at the age of forty-four. The Basser Center for BRCA is the first center devoted to the study of *BRCA*-related cancer. Domchek, the Basser Professor of Oncology, serves as Executive Director of the Center. She recalled the story of how the center came about. "At the request of the Development Office, I got on the phone with Mindy and Jon and talked to them for an hour about the general issues related to these gene mutations. Then, a few weeks later, they contacted us wanting to come down and asked if we would be willing to put together a plan for a center and what that would look like. So we had an initial conversation with them, and then we put together a plan, with an initial $25 million funding request. They funded the $25 million center. Then in 2017, they donated additional $20 million to go into an endowment."

The Basser Center for BRCA has had several major achievements. Domchek has played a key role in the development of poly(ADP ribose) polymerase (PARP) inhibitors for *BRCA*-related cancer. Domchek helmed the trial that led to the first FDA approval of a PARP inhibitor, olaparib, for *BRCA*-associated ovarian cancer.[7] She has been very involved in studies examining PARP inhibitors in *BRCA1/2*-related metastatic breast, pancreatic, and prostate cancer.[8] There are FDA approvals for all of these indications. The Center has also created educational and outreach partnerships for at-risk groups, such as the Philadelphia Jewish community. Angela Bradbury of the Division developed a genetic counseling model using telegenics for communities with limited or no access to these resources. Domchek is very grateful for the philanthropic gift from the Grays. "They're very involved donors who have a real reason that they want to be doing this. They're really committed to the goals. The goals of the center are really to do everything from very basic science to prevention and treatment, and ultimately to change the standard of care for individuals with

BRCA-1 and *-2* mutations so that we're not just recommending preventative surgery."

Under Schuchter's leadership, the Benign Hematology Program has also experienced substantial growth. In 2013, hematologists at Penn and at adjacent CHOP established the Penn-CHOP Blood Center for Patient Care and Discovery. The Penn-CHOP Blood Center is a collaborative program between hematology and laboratory specialists at Penn Medicine and CHOP. Together, they are dedicated to improving the outcomes for both adult and pediatric patients with blood disorders through basic clinical and translational research, and they work to make the transition from pediatric care to adult care seamless for patients and their families. Charles Abrams is Director of the Penn-CHOP Blood Center. In 2016, he served as President of the American Society of Hematology. In an interview when he was President, he was asked what accomplishment in his career he is most proud of. "The accomplishment I am most proud of is one that I couldn't have done alone: developing and serving as director of the Penn-CHOP Blood Center for Patient Care and Discovery at the University of Pennsylvania and Children's Hospital of Philadelphia. This is one of the few blood centers in the United States that provides a full spectrum of care for nonmalignant hematologic disorders. It encompasses adult and pediatric hematology, and there are three major elements: a laboratory, a clinical component, and translational research. The collaboration between our two institutions means that we have become a much stronger, collective program."[9]

Adam Cuker was a Penn Hematology/Oncology fellow from 2006 to 2009. He came to Penn interested in leukemia and bone marrow transplantation, but he recalled, "I was unexpectedly swept off my feet by coagulation."[10] Cuker was supported by

Barbara Konkle's K–12 training grant and earned a master's in translational research at Penn during his fellowship. After joining the faculty in 2009, he became Director of the Penn Comprehensive Hemophilia and Thrombosis Program. This program has about 320 patients with inherited bleeding disorders and more than 800 patients who had experienced thrombosis. Cuker is also Section Leader for Benign Hematology and Associate Director for Clinical Research of the Penn-CHOP Blood Center. Cuker has been actively involved in clinical trials for patients with bleeding disorders. He was a coinvestigator in a seminal CHOP-led research study of adenoviral-based gene therapy for hemophilia B.[11] In addition to Cuker, the clinical benign hematology program includes Farzana Sayani, who developed the sickle cell and thalassemia program, Elaine Chiang in hemophilia, and more recently Allyson Pishko.

Although Schuchter is a clinical and translational researcher, she has been very effective in recruiting world-class fundamental researchers. Through the work of James Hoxie, the Division has demonstrated long-standing excellence in HIV research. To further build on this, Beatrice Hahn and George Shaw were recruited to Penn and the Division in 2011. Hahn and Shaw are international leaders in human and simian immunodeficiency virus research. At the time of their recruitment, Dean Rubinstein stated, "Individually and together, Dr. Hahn and Dr. Shaw will bring additional depth to Penn Medicine in this critical area of science. . . . Their recruitment signals the University's commitment to basic and translational research involving global health pathogens."[12] Both trained as postdoctoral fellows with the virologist Robert Gallo at the National Institutes of Health.[13] When AIDS became a national epidemic in the early 1980s, the isolation and characterization of the responsible virus became the focus of Gallo's laboratory. Hahn and Shaw published the first clones of the HIV virus, which were rapidly deployed to develop diagnostic tests for HIV antibodies.[14] For over three decades, Hahn and Shaw have made major discoveries that have impacted our understanding of immunodeficiency viruses. Hahn's major contributions include identifying the origins of HIV-1 and simian immunodeficiency virus in nonhuman primates. Recently she has focused her research on malaria, which she discovered to have arisen from a cross-species transmission event from African gorillas. Shaw's major contributions include elucidation of the dynamic nature of HIV replication in acute and chronic infection and how HIV escapes immunological control. Of late, he turned his attention to development of a novel simian-human immunodeficiency model of HIV infection in monkeys. For this, he received in 2017 a $16.3 million grant from the National Institute of Allergy and Infectious Diseases to develop a long sought-after HIV vaccine. Both Hahn and Shaw are members of the prestigious National Academy of Medicine, and Hahn was elected to the National Academy of Sciences.

In 2018, Schuchter recruited Ivan Maillard from the University of Michigan to serve the Division as Vice Chief for Research. Maillard, who trained in our fellowship program, investigates the signals regulating the development and function of blood-forming stem cells, focusing on the microenvironment that supports these stem cells. He is responsible for overseeing the research efforts of the Division and is especially interested in mentorship of fellows and junior faculty.

Schuchter is also deeply committed to palliative care. In fact, while serving as Division Chief, she completed a fellowship in palliative care. She recruited to the Division two medical oncologists who were also board certified in palliative care, Anjana Ranganathan and Pallavi Kumar. They served as an important clinical and educational resource for providers in the Division. Schuchter partnered with Lawrence Shulman, ACC Deputy Director of Clinical Services, and Nina O'Connor, Chief of the Palliative Care Program, to implement across the Division the Serious Illness Conversation Program.[15] This is an educational program designed by Susan Block at Harvard to teach providers to have earlier and more effective goals-of-care discussions with patients and families. By the end of 2018, all providers in the Division completed this important training.

Schuchter also has developed the Division's outstanding group of outpatient Advanced Practice Providers led by Suzanne McGettigan. At last count, the Division had over fifty nurse practitioners and physician assistants who are fully integrated into the disease-specific teams and perform independent patient evaluations. In conjunction with Linda Jacobs, ACC's Director of Survivorship, these providers are taking the lead in establishing survivorship clinics for our long-term cancer survivors.

During Schuchter's tenure as Division Chief, the Division has expanded substantially to include other practice sites. Presbyterian Hospital was already part of the Division. When Jack Goldberg retired, Schuchter recruited Evan Alley who had trained in our fellowship to become Chief of Hematology/Oncology at Presbyterian Hospital. When Alley left, another Penn-trained oncologist, Christine Ciunci, assumed the leadership. In 2016, Penn Medicine Cherry Hill opened, significantly increasing the patient capacity both in examination rooms and in the infusion suite. To staff this increased capacity, a private practice group led by our former fellow Richard Greenberg joined the Division. In addition, Penn opened an outpatient facility in Valley Forge, Pennsylvania. Schuchter hired two full-time hematologists/oncologists, Tracey D'Entremont, a former Penn fellow, and John Kosteva. Most recently, Penn Medicine Radnor has opened a new state-of-the-art medical building with much-expanded cancer-related services.

With changes in medical reimbursement, private practice hematology/oncology groups had to confront significant financial challenges. Nationally, many private practice groups joined larger, often academic organizations. Arthur Staddon of Pennsylvania Hematology/Oncology group, who practiced at Pennsylvania Hospital, stated that during the practice's prime, it used the profits made from drugs to fund the clinical research efforts of the group. He recalled, "We covered all the research costs ourselves. We did trials because we thought it was important for either the scientific point or for our patients." He then added, "The economics of private practice were such that payments kept going lower and the costs for the drugs kept going up."[16] Staddon knew that they could not continue business as usual.

In 2013, the physicians of Pennsylvania Hematology/Oncology became full-time faculty of the Division. This group of hematologists/oncologists is led by David Mintzer. Patricia Ford has been instrumental in the development of a bloodless surgery program at Pennsylvania Hospital, developed for patients who are Jehovah's Witnesses. Staddon recently retired. In announcing his retirement, Schuchter wrote, "Please join me in congratulating Dr. Arthur 'Chip' Staddon on his recent retirement from Penn Medicine. He has had a truly remarkable career. Amazingly, Chip was chief resident at HUP fifty years ago. As part of his retirement celebration, Chip was also honored this week by being awarded the 2018 Good Samaritan Award from Pennsylvania Hospital. Since 1985, the Good Samaritan Award has been given to an individual who has provided exemplary volunteer leadership and support with a spirit of generosity and caring for Pennsylvania Hospital."[17]

Dennis Berman joined our fellowship program in 1981. After two years, he left the fellowship to start a private practice in hematology/oncology in West Chester. At the time, there was no hematology/oncology service in this part of suburban Philadelphia. He recalled, "At the end of my first year, I met the pathologist Hugh Bonner. We got to be friends, and Hugh finally coerced me to come out and manage the tumor conference on Wednesday morning at Chester County Hospital. This is the beginning of my second year of fellowship. Then they started bringing patients out and wanted me to see them after tumor conference. I called Buz and Buz said, 'Yes. Do it! Jane Alavi will be your backup attending.' I started seeing six, eight new patients on the Wednesday that I came out there. By the end of my second year of my fellowship I was so busy with the clinical practice I had to make a decision to either stop doing that and just do a third year of research or leave."[18] So he left the fellowship after two years and built a superb private practice hematology/oncology group at West Chester. Many of its providers graduated from our fellowship program, including Will Luginbuhl, Maureen Hewitt, and James "Mac" Patterson.

In 2013, Chester County Hospital joined Penn Medicine. Due to financial issues similar to those that confronted the Pennsylvania Hospital group, it became clear to Berman that his group would need to become part of a larger entity. In 2016, the members of his private practice group became full-time members of the

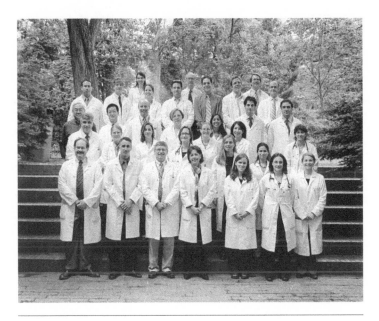

Figure 5. Division, 2008. Division Chief Lynn Schuchter is in the front row, fourth from left.

Division. Presently, there are ten full-time Hematology/Oncology providers at West Chester. More recently, Lancaster General Hospital and the Princeton Health Care System became part of Penn Medicine. It is anticipated that the Division will become even larger (and more complex) as these centers are further integrated into the health system.

ELEVEN

Immunotherapy Comes of Age

As a fellow, I remember reading case reports of patients with metastatic renal cell carcinoma whose metastases regressed after removal of the kidney. It was felt that this was an immunologically mediated event. As a resident, I read with amazement Stephen Rosenberg's *New England Journal of Medicine* paper showing that patients with metastatic melanoma could enter durable remissions when treated with high-dose interleukin-2 (IL-2) and tumor-infiltrating lymphocytes.[1] When there was early enthusiasm for expanding research in high-dose IL-2 therapy, the NCI asked comprehensive cancer centers such as Penn to join a multi-center clinical trial of high-dose IL-2 in patients with metastatic melanoma or renal cell cancer. As the most junior member of the Division, Kevin Fox was charged with being principal investigator on this trial. Patients were electively admitted to the medical intensive care unit and treated with high-dose IL-2. From 1988 to 1989, eighteen patients were treated at Penn. Fox recalls tremendous toxicity, putting the patient into what looked like a state of septic shock, and little benefit. "That's a period of my life I would rather forget," Fox told me.[2] When I arrived at Penn in 1990, high-dose IL-2 had been abandoned.

During my early years on the faculty, I remember consulting on a male patient in his mid-thirties who had a painful tooth extracted, and the dentist sent the tooth to pathology. The pathologist identified malignant cells, and on further investigation the patient was found to have a large kidney mass, multiple bone lesions, and multiple lung metastases. He underwent nephrectomy, and pathologic results demonstrated renal clear cell carcinoma. He had no symptoms, was big and strong, and rode a Harley Davidson motorcycle. I discussed with him the limited options available (at that time) and discussed a trial of high-dose IL-2 being performed at the NCI. The patient jumped at this opportunity, and for several months I did not see or hear from him. About six months later, he returned to see me as his disease had progressed, and he had been taken off the protocol. I asked him about his experience with this treatment and was startled when he told me that being on hemodialysis and a ventilator for a few days was not as bad as he thought it might be. He was describing the life-threatening toxicity associated with high-dose IL-2. Immunotherapy was simply not ready for prime time.

I first met Robert Vonderheide soon after he arrived at Penn in 2001. Like many newly arrived faculty, he reached out to learn more about what I did at Penn and whether there were opportunities for collaboration. He was young, energetic, and very enthusiastic. His passion for immunological approaches to cancer therapy was intoxicating but at the time seemed a bit futuristic. He came to Penn at a time when chemotherapy was still the primary modality for systemically treating cancer and targeted therapy was just starting to be developed in clinical trials. Vonderheide believed that immunotherapy was the future of cancer treatment and that Penn would lead the way. We did not know how right he was.

Vonderheide focused much of his work on a protein called CD40. This protein is found on the surface of antigen-presenting cells such as macrophages. These are the cells that present a protein fragment to the T cell to initiate an immune response. Activation of CD40 is a key regulatory step for the development of T cell–dependent antitumor immunity. Vonderheide initially performed a phase I trial of a monoclonal antibody that targets CD40 (a so-called CD40 agonist).[3] Subsequently, he and his postdoctoral fellow Gregory L. Beatty (who trained in our Hematology/Oncology fellowship program and is now an Associate Professor of Medicine in our Division) hypothesized that in a disease like pancreatic ductal carcinoma, known to be immunosuppressive, treatment with a CD40 agonist would result in activation of tumor-specific immune T cells. They combined the CD40 agonist with the standard pancreatic cancer chemotherapy drug gemcitabine and demonstrated that patients with metastatic pancreatic cancer could benefit from this combination. They then set out to determine why. They reproduced the human clinical trial in a genetically engineered mouse model of pancreatic ductal carcinoma. They again noted an antitumor effect of this combination but then observed something quite unexpected. Tumor regression required CD40-activated macrophages but not T cell activation or gemcitabine treatment. They demonstrated that in fact these activated macrophages themselves infiltrated tumors, were tumoricidal in and of themselves, and resulted in the depletion of tumor stroma or surrounding tissue. Vonderheide and Beatty discovered a previously unknown approach to target immunosuppressive tumors.[4] It is this kind of innovative and highly translational research, as

well as his outstanding mentorship skills, that established Vonderheide as one of the international leaders in the field of cancer
immunotherapy.

The development of immune checkpoint inhibitors represents
one of the most important recent breakthroughs in cancer treatment. The immune system has checkpoints that are analogous to a
brake on the system. Tumor cells use these checkpoints to neutral-
ize a patient's immune system. Checkpoint inhibitors are monoclonal antibodies directed against the proteins on the surface of the
T cell (such as CTLA4 and PD-1) or tumor cell (such as PD-L1)
responsible for the checkpoint. By inhibiting the brakes on the
immune system, antitumor immunity can awaken, resulting in
tumor regression.

Faculty in the Hematology/Oncology Division have played a
major role in the clinical development of these inhibitors. Tara
Mitchell and colleagues have extensively evaluated these agents in
melanoma.[5] Checkpoint inhibitors have also played a major role
in the treatment of non–small cell lung cancer, and the thoracic
group led by Corey Langer has had an active role in the development of these agents.[6]

Immune checkpoint inhibitors have also had a major impact
in metastatic bladder cancer. While these patients can respond to
platinum-based chemotherapy, most subsequently progress and
die of their disease. The treatment of these patients was considered an unmet need and thus a fruitful area of research for a junior
faculty member to focus on. During the early years of my career,
I was principal investigator on several trials of novel cytotoxic
agents, such as paclitaxel and vinflunine in patients with metastatic bladder cancer whose disease had progressed after platinum-
based chemotherapy. Although these trials resulted in several
publications to add to my CV—always important for a junior

faculty member building a career—most were "negative trials," meaning the treatment did not benefit patients.

At our annual ASCO meeting in 2015, the early results of using the anti-PD-L1 agent atezolizumab and the anti-PD-1 monoclonal antibody pembrolizumab in metastatic bladder cancer were presented. These were so-called bucket trials in which patients with a variety of tumor types were treated with these agents. I was struck by the results. About a third of patients with metastatic bladder cancer, all of whom had their tumors grow despite chemotherapy, experienced favorable responses to this therapy, some of which were durable. I left the meeting invigorated, knowing that we needed to get access to these drugs for our patients.

We subsequently participated in a Merck-sponsored clinical trial known as KEYNOTE 45.[7] In this trial, patients with metastatic bladder cancer who had previously received platinum-based chemotherapy were randomly assigned to receive second-line chemotherapy with an agent such a docetaxel or to receive the experimental agent pembrolizumab. A memorable patient was an eighty-year-old woman with metastatic bladder cancer who had received platinum-based chemotherapy and whose disease had progressed. She had very extensive lung metastases, so extensive that she was short of breath at rest and required oxygen. She was randomly assigned to the pembrolizumab arm, and after three cycles her symptoms started to improve, although her CT scan results did not. However, after six cycles she was off oxygen, had resumed normal activity, and had a marked regression in her lung metastases. I had never seen anything quite like this before. Six months later she was traveling with her family in Italy. She ultimately succumbed to her disease, but truly had a remarkable response to therapy with virtually no side effects. Most of the patients who were randomly assigned to chemotherapy did not benefit, while about 20 percent of the patients receiving pembrolizumab experienced long-term disease control. Based on this trial, the FDA approved pembrolizumab for the second-line treatment of patients with platinum-refractory metastatic bladder cancer. Prior to this, the last drug to be approved for metastatic bladder cancer was cisplatin in 1978.

In April 2016, the Parker Foundation announced a $250 million grant to establish the Parker Institute for Cancer Immunotherapy. On their website the Parker Institute states, "For decades, entrenched infrastructure barriers have slowed progress in the fight against cancer and the development of potent immunotherapies. The Parker Institute breaks down these barriers. The result is a groundbreaking new research and intellectual property model that builds collaboration between researchers, nonprofits and industry all working together to get treatments to patients faster."[8] The ACC was one of the institutions selected to join this institute. In 2016, Gerald Linette was recruited to the Hematology/ Oncology Division to serve as the Medical Director of the Parker Institute for Cancer Immunotherapy at the Perelman School of Medicine at the University of Pennsylvania. Linette's primary interest is the development of cellular immunotherapies for melanoma and other solid tumors. His laboratory research is focused on human tumor neoantigen discovery, a potential key to optimizing immunotherapy for cancer.

Cancer immunotherapy with checkpoint inhibitors has become standard treatment for many types of cancer. We are still learning how to select the patients most likely to benefit and how to optimize the effectiveness of this approach, but the research is rapidly advancing. As oncologists and hematologists, we have by necessity needed to become immunologists, very much to our patients' benefit. Although most patients tolerate these treatments well, patients can develop severe immune-mediated side effects, such as colitis, pituitary gland dysfunction, and diabetes, among other toxicities. This notwithstanding, the development of immune checkpoint inhibitors represents an important advance in cancer medicine.

Vonderheide was right when he predicted that immunotherapy would play a central role in oncology and that Penn would lead the way. In July 2017, he was named Director of the ACC. He succeeded Chi Van Dang who, having served as ACC Director since 2011, resigned to become Scientific Director of the Ludwig Institute. Vonderheide's appointment as Director was embraced by the Hematology/Oncology faculty given his commitment to translational research and clinical trials. In 2020, Vonderheide submitted the competitive renewal of our CCSG, and this grant application was rated "exceptional" by the NCI. Under his leadership, Penn will remain one of the top centers in the country for innovative, investigator-initiated cancer clinical trials.

TWELVE

A Revolutionary Treatment

Carl June is perhaps the most celebrated of the scientists that Craig Thompson and John Glick recruited to the AFCRI. June is the Richard W. Vague Professor in Immunotherapy in the Department of Pathology and Laboratory Medicine and Director of Penn's Center for Cellular Immunotherapies. He trained in bone marrow transplantation at the Fred Hutchinson Cancer Research Center when Thompson was there. Before coming to Penn in 1999, June was at the Uniformed Services University/Naval Medical Research Institute, where he and colleagues made a major discovery: the CD28 molecule plays a central role in T cell biology.[1] June's landmark contribution to the field of oncology is the development of chimeric antigen receptor T cell (CAR-T) therapy. On the surface of all cells is an array of proteins, some quite specific to the cell type. The basic premise of the approach is that T cells, which are immune cells, can be harvested from the peripheral blood of a patient and taken to the laboratory, where they are genetically modified to express a specific receptor that binds to a specific protein on the surface of a tumor cell (and often its normal counterpart). These genetically modified T cells are then reinfused into the patient. June initially used this approach to treat HIV/AIDS and demonstrated that the reinfused cells could engraft and persist for years.[2] He then turned his attention to using CAR-T therapy to eradicate cancer. The CD19 molecule is expressed on the surface of normal B cells and B cell neoplasms, such as chronic lymphocytic leukemia and certain forms of acute lymphoblastic leukemia and non-Hodgkin's lymphoma. June developed CAR-T 19 therapy, and after testing it in animal models wanted to bring this approach to human patients. He needed a partner on the clinical side, and he reached out to David Porter.

Porter was the ideal collaborator. He had built the allogeneic stem cell transplant program at Penn. As a fellow at Harvard, he performed studies of allogeneic donor T cell infusions for relapsed leukemia and was one of the first to demonstrate the benefit of this immunological approach. CAR-T therapy was a logical extension of his previous work. He knew of the interesting laboratory work that was happening in the June laboratory, where novel immunotherapy such as genetically modified T cell therapies were being developed in animal models. During 2009, Porter spent a six-month sabbatical learning about CAR-T and immunology. He attended the June laboratory meetings and met with June and other members of his lab. He then designed and wrote the first Penn pilot trial of CAR-T 19 therapy for refractory chronic lymphocytic leukemia (CLL).

Porter treated his first patient with CAR-T 19 in 2010. He reported his preliminary results in the *New England Journal of Medicine* in 2011[3] and the mature results in *Science and Translational Medicine* in 2015.[4] Of fourteen patients with refractory

CLL treated with CAR-T 19, eight responded and four went into durable complete remissions. In the first two patients who achieved a complete remission, the CAR-T 19 cells persisted and were functional more than four years after treatment. These results were unprecedented.

Porter was appointed Director of the newly formed Cell Therapy and Transplant (CTT) program within the ACC. The CTT program encompasses both clinical and experimental cellular therapies that include bone marrow transplant, CAR-T, and other immune therapies. The mission of CTT is to support the ACC, the Division of Hematology/Oncology, and the Center for Cellular Immunotherapy to provide the most effective and innovative cellular therapies to as many patients in need as safely as possible. Alison Loren, who became Director of Blood and Marrow Transplantation, told me, "The truth is David Porter is a remarkable innovator in hematology and has had, by my count, three world-changing contributions. He was one of the early pioneers of donor lymphocyte therapy. He was one the early pioneers of reduced intensity transplant. And obviously CAR-T. He's really changed the world."[5]

The promise of CAR-T therapy led to a partnership between Penn and Novartis, which signed a global collaboration and licensing agreement in 2012 to further research, develop, and commercialize CAR-T therapies to treat cancer. As part of their agreement, Penn and Novartis constructed a first-of-its-kind Center for Advanced Cellular Therapeutics on the Penn campus that is devoted to the discovery, development, and manufacturing of adoptive T cell immunotherapies through a joint research and development program led by scientists and clinicians from Penn, Novartis, and the Novartis Institutes for Biomedical Research. Novartis committed $20 million to the project, covering the bulk of the center's construction costs.

Given the success of CAR-T 19 therapy in CLL, June and colleagues next targeted refractory acute B cell leukemia in children and adults. Stephen Grupp and his mentee Shannon Maude led the clinical efforts at CHOP. Porter's junior colleague and a former Hematology/Oncology fellow, Noelle Frey, led the team at HUP. In October 2014, they reported the results in the first thirty children and adults who were treated.[6] Remarkably, 90 percent of these patients achieved complete remission. The major toxicity of this trial was cytokine-release syndrome (CRS), a potentially life-threatening toxicity caused by immune activation. CRS is characterized by fever, low blood pressure, and respiratory issues. The investigators determined that CRS was mediated through release of interleukin-6 (IL-6), and they successfully used the anti-IL-6 receptor antibody tocilizumab to reverse this condition.[7]

Based on these promising results, a multicenter trial of sixty-three pediatric and young adults (all aged twenty-five years or younger) with relapsed or refractory acute lymphocytic leukemia (ALL) was performed. The complete remission rate with CAR-T 19 therapy was 83 percent.[8] On August 30, 2017, the FDA approved CAR-T 19, now called tisagenlecleucel (Kymriah, Novartis Pharmaceuticals Corporation), for pediatric and young adult patients with relapsed or refractory ALL. This treatment represents the first gene therapy approved by the FDA. Given this age of social media, it was only appropriate that Penn/CHOP faculty, staff, patients, families, and friends celebrated this remarkable achievement with a "flash mob" celebration held in the lobby of the Perelman Center for Advanced Medicine. At the celebration, Vonderheide spoke: "Today's landmark decision by the FDA to approve Kymriah represents two decades of investment and perseverance by Penn's Abramson Cancer Center and our partners CHOP and Novartis. The approval of this revolutionary therapy transforms care and provides a new option for patients whose leukemia is no longer responding to standard approaches."[9]

The results of this revolutionary research are unprecedented and have attracted worldwide attention. Emily Whitehead was six years old and had refractory ALL and limited options when she enrolled in the initial phase I trial of CAR-T 19. She has been in remission since May 2012. Her story has been widely publicized both in the press and on television. Emily has become the face of CAR-T, and she and her parents are committed to helping other patients with cancer. The Emily Whitehead Foundation's mission is "to raise awareness and funding for innovative childhood cancer treatments, such as immunotherapy, that will improve survival rates and quality of life."[10]

For his groundbreaking research, June was named on *Time*'s listing of the 100 Most Influential People of 2018. His tribute was written by Emily: "I was a fun and energetic child. Then I spent two years in a hospital getting cancer treatment, but it wasn't working for me. That's when my parents and I learned about an experimental treatment, called T cell, that would train my immune system to fight my cancer; it hadn't been tried on a pediatric patient before. My parents believed that this was the right choice for me, and we transferred to the Children's Hospital of Philadelphia to enter the trial. After getting the treatment, I went into a 14-day coma and awakened on my seventh birthday. But the treatment had worked! We later learned that Dr. Carl June's research had created this treatment. Dr. June saved my life and had a huge impact on my family. Without him, I wouldn't be here today writing this—and my parents and I wouldn't be helping other kids beat cancer. Dr. June is my hero! He saved my family."[11]

While the groundbreaking research in leukemia was ongoing, Stephen Schuster turned his attention to B cell non-Hodgkin's lymphoma since this type of cancer also expresses on the cell surface the antigen CD19. He led a trial of tisagenlecleucel in patients with relapsed or refractory diffuse large B cell lymphoma (DLBCL) or follicular lymphoma. Eighteen of twenty-eight adult patients responded favorably to this treatment. With over two years of follow-up, 86 percent of the patients with DLBCL who responded and 89 percent of the patients with follicular lymphoma who responded experienced sustained remissions.[12] These promising results led to a multicenter phase 2 trial of tisagenlecleucel in patients with relapsed or refractory DLBCL. In sixty-eight patients, the overall response rate was 50 percent, with a complete response rate of 32 percent. On May 1, 2018, the FDA approved tisagenlecleucel for adult patients with relapsed or refractory large B cell lymphoma after two or more lines of systemic therapy, including DLBCL not otherwise specified, high-grade B cell lymphoma, and DLBCL arising from follicular lymphoma. Not unexpectedly, this historic event was celebrated by a second "flash mob" celebration in the PCAM lobby orchestrated by Vonderheide. Reflecting on this remarkable achievement, Schuster said, "Working on this has been the best experience of my professional life. And we're going to keep making it better at Penn."[13]

EPILOGUE

I finished the first draft of this manuscript as I completed my three-month sabbatical in September 2018. I circulated it to several colleagues for suggestions and made revisions. I started to look into options for publishing, but life as a busy clinical oncologist took precedent. Every few months I would pull the manuscript out and tinker a bit, but I must admit that I lost momentum on the project. Then in March 2020, the COVID-19 pandemic hit. As of this writing, over 700,000 Americans have died from this deadly virus. We have all learned that one never knows what tomorrow will bring. This led me to feel some urgency to get this manuscript completed and published. In addition, the Division of Hematology/Oncology will celebrate its fiftieth anniversary in 2022. To commemorate this important event, I was determined to get this history updated and into print. However, given the unprecedented nature of the COVID-19 pandemic, I felt it was important to conclude with how this event impacted the Division and how the Division responded.

Before discussing the pandemic, it is important to note three historic events that have transpired over the past year (reviewed in chronological order). First, on April 15, 2020, our great benefactor Madlyn Abramson passed away. Together with her husband, Leonard, Madlyn gave more than $140 million to support the Abramson Cancer Center. With her generosity and vision, the Division and the Cancer Center have attained an unprecedented level of excellence in cancer care, clinical trials, and cancer immunotherapy. Former ACC Director John Glick reflected, "Never could I be more proud that the Abramson Cancer Center bears the name of Madlyn, who has done so much to bring healing, compassion, and hope to people facing cancer. Her philanthropy has simply been transformational in the care of patients with cancer. We will all miss her dearly." Current ACC Director Robert Vonderheide added, "The reputation we enjoy today as one of the nation's preeminent cancer centers has been built on the strong foundation that Madlyn laid. The exciting progress we've made in pursuit of curing cancer unites us every day to do more for our patients here in the Abramson Cancer Center and across the world, and we have Madlyn, together with her husband, Leonard, to thank for the vision that set us on this path."[1]

The second significant event was the retirement of a legend. On May 19, 2021, Larry Jameson, Dean of the School of Medicine, and Kevin Mahoney, CEO of UPHS, sent out this email to the Penn Medicine community: "We write to announce that after nearly five decades of unsurpassed leadership and impact at Penn Medicine, John H. Glick, MD, Professor of Medicine and the Madlyn & Leonard Abramson Professor of Clinical Oncology, will retire at the end of the academic year."[2] To commemorate this historic event, Lynn Schuchter asked the Division's faculty to send her personal sentiments and recollections about Glick that she would collate into a book for him. On June 23, 2021, the Division held a retirement celebration to honor Glick. Several of these recollections were read, and colleagues reflected on his impact (via ZOOM given the ongoing pandemic). The following is what I wrote and read, which I believe truly reflects the character of this great man: "During my early years on the faculty, John was a wonderful mentor, frequently checking in and making sure that I was doing well both in and out of work. However, he never let me forget who was ultimately in charge. I recall one Saturday as a junior faculty member when he invited me to play golf at his club. I was nervous to start, but he only made things worse. On one tee as I was addressing the ball getting ready to hit my drive, John asked, 'So David, how is your promotion to Associate Professor coming along? I hear getting promoted is getting tougher these days.' Needless to say, I became unglued and duck-hooked my drive into the woods. He then reminded me that I could hit another drive, but I needed to take a penalty stroke. No mulligans when you play golf with John! In 1999, our son Luke was diagnosed with autism. This was a very difficult time, and my distress must have been apparent when John called me into his office and asked me what was wrong. I told him about Luke's diagnosis, and as he listened, I could see tears in his eyes. He invited Annie and me over to his house the next day for dinner. He and Jane listened to the challenges that we were facing. John told me that he and Penn were going to help get us through this difficult time. He helped us develop a plan moving forward and gave us hope and encouragement. He has been there for us ever since. My extreme loyalty to the Division, Cancer Center, and Penn is in large part a result of John's exceptional mentorship and friendship."

Finally, on June 20, 2021, our friend and colleague Joel Bennett passed away. Charles Abrams delivered this sad news to us and in his announcement described Bennett's seminal research and accomplishments. He then continued, "But there was so much more to Joel than him being an accomplished NIH-funded physician scientist. Joel was truly a renaissance man, who while being the consummate academician always had a terrific sense of grace, life, and whimsy. He was one of a kind, and he approached everything with exceptional thought and care. Joel tirelessly and without fail was there to lend a hand and bolster our spirits when things got difficult. He never lost his sense of humor and wit, even in the darkest of times. Most importantly, Joel was a cherished friend and colleague who has touched our lives and who shall never be forgotten."[3]

During the past year, the Division has confronted unprecedented challenges because of the COVID-19 pandemic. However, Schuchter's leadership was never more apparent as she steered the great vessel that is the Division through the uncharted waters that were the pandemic. Beginning in March 2020, when cases began to be reported in the Philadelphia region, she led daily huddles to review unfolding events and determine how the Division would respond. From addressing providers' concerns about how to safely practice cancer medicine through the rapid incorporation of telemedicine into our practice and ultimately to the rollout of the vaccine to our patients and providers, Schuchter has shone. Her Friday-afternoon COVID update emails to the Division were both informational and inspiring. She never failed to highlight the successes of her faculty during this difficult time, from important publications and honors to more personal life events, such as birth announcements complete with photographs. These emails

often included a touch of humor and good cheer, always remind-
ing us that indeed we would get through these difficult times.

Following Schuchter's example, the Division's faculty responded
to the pandemic with remarkable enthusiasm and productivity,
not only in the clinic but through cutting-edge research. Ravi
Amaravadi and colleagues reported a double-blind, randomized,
clinical trial examining whether preexposure prophylaxis with
the autophagy inhibitor hydroxychloroquine in hospital-based
health care workers prevented transmission of SARS-CoV-2. Although the trial did not demonstrate clinical benefit of hydroxychloroquine, the rapidity and efficiency of developing, completing,
and reporting this innovative research protocol was unprecedented.[4] Alexander Huang and colleagues reported an important
study in patients with cancer who had been hospitalized for
COVID-19 infection. They demonstrated that patients with hematologic malignancies had a higher mortality than those with
solid tumors. They then sought to understand why by studying
the immunologic response to SARS-CoV-2. They demonstrated
that patients with solid tumors and patients without cancer had
a similar immune response during acute COVID-19 infection.
However, patients with hematologic malignancies had impaired
B cell function and SARS-CoV-2-specific antibody response.
They additionally demonstrated that patients with hematologic
malignancies who had a greater number of CD8 T cells had improved survival. This suggested that CD8 T cells might compen-
sate when humoral immunity is deficient.[5]

When the pandemic began, caring for patients with cancer was
uncharted territory. Balancing the risk of infection against the
risk of cancer progression was an unprecedented challenge. Division faculty helped to define how to optimally care for these patients
in the midst of the COVID-19 pandemic. Studies subsequently

demonstrated the negative impact of delaying cancer care because of COVID-19. Lova Sun and colleagues demonstrated that patients with cancer receiving care in an outpatient treatment center that had adopted aggressive mitigation measures had a SARS-CoV-2 seroconversion rate of 0 percent during the course of receiving outpatient treatment, highlighting that cancer care can be delivered safely even at the height of a pandemic.[6] Aditi Singh and colleagues published widely cited guidelines for caring for patients with lung cancer during the pandemic. They recommended that general principles of lung cancer management should be followed in most cases, despite the pandemic.[7] Benign hematology faculty played an important role in helping to understand why patients with COVID-19 experienced thrombosis and what should be done about this. Adam Cuker led an ASH guideline committee to establish best practices for the use of anticoagulation in thromboprophylaxis in patients with COVID-19.[8] Faculty also represented the Division on several national and international guidelines committees in leukemia (Keith Pratz and Selina Luger),[9] myeloma (Edward Stadtmauer),[10] and CAR-T (David Porter).[11]

On September 30, 2020, at the height of the pandemic, Vonderheide and the ACC sponsored a continuing medical education webinar entitled "COVID-19 and Cancer" in which the complexities of providing cancer care during the COVID-19 pandemic were discussed. Division faculty spoke about principles of cancer care during COVID-19 and presented original research. This evening program was highlighted by a keynote address from Anthony Fauci, Director of the National Institute of Allergy and Infectious Diseases. The evening was a memorable moment of brightness during a dark stretch of time.

Because of COVID-19 vaccination, life in the Division is slowly but surely returning to normal. We are now seeing most of our patients in the clinics rather than through telemedicine. Our daily, then weekly, then monthly COVID-19 huddles are no longer needed, as issues related to COVID-19 are now discussed in our other regular meetings. We are running into each other again in our offices, clinics, and inpatient floors. During the COVID-19 pandemic, we watched in awe as the Pavilion rose. This new, innovative, inpatient hospital due to open in October 2021 will house over 500 private patient rooms, an expanded emergency department, and 47 operating rooms in a 1.5-million-square-foot, 17-story facility across from the Hospital of the University of Pennsylvania and adjacent to the Perelman Center for Advanced Medicine.[12] Division faculty look forward to the opportunity to care for our patients in such an outstanding setting.

—————

As I reflect on the fifty-year history of the Division, there are certain themes that seem evident though the years. Innovative and rigorous scientific inquiry has not only advanced medical discovery; it has also been translated into important gains for our patients. A steadfast commitment to clinical excellence in benign and malignant hematology and solid tumor oncology offers our patients the most advanced and compassionate care available. Philanthropy has played an important role in the Division's success, as evidenced by many transformative gifts throughout the years. Most importantly, the Division has benefited from remarkable leadership since its founding. Buz Cooper integrated hematology and oncology at Penn and established the Cancer Center. Sandy Shattil expanded outstanding fundamental research in the Division. Stephen Emerson innovatively developed solid tumor oncology and transformed malignant hematology and bone marrow transplant. Lynn Schuchter led tremendous expansion of the Division, with the integration of Hematology/Oncology across several

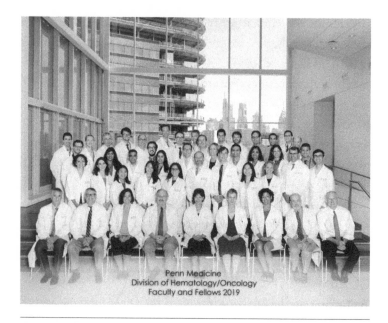

Penn Medicine
Division of Hematology/Oncology
Faculty and Fellows 2019

Figure 6. Division, 2019. Division Chief Lynn Schuchter is in the front row, fifth from left.

Penn hospitals. In addition, she shepherded the Division through the unprecedented COVID-19 pandemic. Through these four eras, John Glick remained an anchor, from leading the Cancer Center for over two decades to establishing the AFCRI to helping to make PCAM a reality.

On June 16, 2021, at the Division's monthly faculty meeting, Schuchter announced her plans to step down as Division Chief by June 30, 2022. In a follow-up email announcement to the Division, she wrote, "You have given me the greatest gift in allowing me to lead one of the very top Hematology/Oncology Divisions in the country. You are all making a difference, every day, and I could not be prouder of this division and all that we have achieved together during this transformational time for our field."[13] Vonderheide will lead a national search committee to recruit her replacement. As we celebrate our fiftieth anniversary in 2022, we will raise a glass to honor the many remarkable members of our Division who have contributed so much. We will also toast our future division chief and the next chapter of this remarkable story that is Penn's Division of Hematology/Oncology.

Current Faculty of the Division of Hematology/Oncology (as of July 2021)

Name	Title	Location	Specialty (if applicable)
Erin O. Aakhus, MD	Program Director, Hematology/Oncology Fellowship Program	HUP/VA	Thoracic/Head and Neck
	Assistant Professor of Clinical Medicine		
Charles S. Abrams, MD	Vice Chair for Research and Chief Scientific Officer, Department of Medicine	HUP	Benign Hematology/ Fundamental Research
	Director, PENN-CHOP Blood Center for Patient Care and Discovery		
	Professor of Medicine in Pathology and Laboratory Medicine		
	Francis C. Wood Professor*		

(Continued)

Name	Title	Location	Specialty (if applicable)
Sandra Susanibar Adaniya, MD	Assistant Professor of Medicine at the Hospital of the University of Pennsylvania	HUP	Myeloma
Charu Aggarwal, MD, MPH	Leslye M. Heisler Associate Professor for Lung Cancer Excellence*	HUP	Thoracic
Daniel Altman, MD	Clinical Associate in Medicine	CCH	
Ravi K. Amaravadi, MD	Co-Leader of the Cancer Therapeutics Program, Abramson Cancer Center	HUP	Melanoma/ Developmental Therapeutics
	Associate Professor of Medicine at the Hospital of the University of Pennsylvania		
Daria V. Babushok, MD, PhD	Assistant Professor of Pediatrics	HUP	Hematologic Malignancies/ Fundamental Research
	Assistant Professor of Medicine		
Stephen Bagley, MD, MSCE	Assistant Professor of Neurosurgery	HUP	Neuro-oncology
	Assistant Professor of Medicine at the Hospital of the University of Pennsylvania		
Stefan Barta, MD, MS, MRCPCUK	Director, T-Cell Lymphoma Program	HUP	Lymphoma
	Executive Officer, AIDS Malignancy Consortium		
	Associate Professor of Clinical Medicine		
Douglas F. Beach, MD	Director, CREP/Breast and Ovarian Cancer Program (PAH)	PAH	

Name	Title	Location	Specialty (if applicable)
	Associate Program Director, Internal Medicine Residency (PAH)		
	Clinical Assistant Professor of Medicine		
Gregory L. Beatty, MD, PhD	Director, Clinical and Translational Research, Penn Pancreatic Cancer Research Center	HUP	GI/Fundamental Research
	Associate Professor of Medicine		
Saveri Bhattacharya, DO	Assistant Professor of Clinical Medicine	HUP	Breast
Angela R. Bradbury, MD	Associate Professor of Medicine at the Hospital of the University of Pennsylvania	HUP	Breast/Cancer Genetics
	Associate Professor of Medical Ethics and Health Policy		
Lawrence F. Brass, MD, PhD	Professor of Pharmacology	HUP	Benign Hematology/ Fundamental Research
	Professor of Medicine		
Ximena Jordan Bruno, MD	Assistant Professor of Clinical Medicine	HUP	Leukemia
Mehar Burki, MD	Clinical Associate in Medicine	CCH	
Erica Carpenter, MBA, PhD	Research Assistant Professor of Medicine	HUP	Fundamental Research
	Assistant Professor of Pathology and Laboratory Medicine		
Martin P. Carroll, MD	Associate Professor of Medicine	HUP/VA	Leukemia/Fundamental Research
Elaine Y. Chiang, MD	Associate Professor of Clinical Medicine	HUP	Benign Hematology

(Continued)

Name	Title	Location	Specialty (if applicable)
Elise A. Chong, MD	Assistant Professor of Medicine at the Hospital of the University of Pennsylvania	HUP	Lymphoma
Christine A. Ciunci, MD, MSCE	Section Chief, Hematology/Oncology, Penn Presbyterian Medical Center	PPMC	Thoracic
	Physician Lead, Cancer Service Line, Penn Presbyterian Medical Center		
	Assistant Professor of Clinical Medicine		
Amy S. Clark, MD, MSCE	Deputy Director, Breast Cancer Clinical Trials	HUP	Breast
	Assistant Professor of Medicine at the Hospital of the University of Pennsylvania		
Adam D. Cohen, MD	Director, Myeloma Immunotherapy	HUP	Myeloma
	Associate Professor of Medicine at the Hospital of the University of Pennsylvania		
Justine V. Cohen, DO	Clinical Assistant Professor of Medicine	PAH	
Roger B. Cohen, MD	Associate Director of Clinical Research, Abramson Cancer Center	HUP	Thoracic/Head and Neck
	Associate Director, Hematology/Oncology Fellowship Program		
	Professor of Medicine at the Hospital of the University of Pennsylvania		
Michael R. Costello, MD	Clinical Associate of Medicine	CCH	

Name	Title	Location	Specialty (if applicable)
Adam C. Cuker, MD, MS	Director, Penn Comprehensive and Hemophilia Thrombosis Program	HUP	Benign Hematology
	Assistant Director, Hematology/Oncology Fellowship Program		
	Clinical Director, Penn Blood Disorders Center, University of Pennsylvania		
	Section Chief, Benign Hematology		
	Associate Professor of Medicine in Pathology and Laboratory Medicine		
	Associate Professor of Medicine at the Hospital of the University of Pennsylvania		
Nevena Damjanov, MD	Section Chief Hematology/ Oncology, VA Medical Center	VA/ PPMC	GI
	Director of Gastrointestinal Oncology, Abramson Cancer Center, Penn Presbyterian Medical Center		
	Professor of Clinical Medicine		
Christopher A. D'Avella, MD	Assistant Professor of Clinical Medicine	PPMC	
Angela DeMichele, MD, MSCE	Co-Leader, Breast Cancer Research Program	HUP	Breast
	Director, Breast Cancer Clinical Trials Unit		
	Co-Director, 2-PREVENT Breast Cancer Translational Research Center		
	Alan and Jill Miller Professor in Breast Cancer Excellence*		

(*Continued*)

Name	Title	Location	Specialty (if applicable)
Tracy S. d'Entremont, MD	Director of Oncology Services, Abramson Cancer Center at Valley Forge	VF	
	Clinical Assistant Professor of Medicine		
Arati Desai, MD	Assistant Professor of Neurosurgery	HUP	Neuro-oncology
	Assistant Professor of Clinical Medicine		
Mark Diamond, MD, PhD	Instructor A of Medicine	HUP	Melanoma
Susan M. Domchek, MD	Executive Director, Basser Center for BRCA	HUP	Breast/Cancer Genetics
	Director, MacDonald Women's Cancer Risk Evaluation Center		
	Basser Professor in Oncology*		
Jennifer R. Eads, MD	Physician Lead GI Clinical Research	HUP	GI
	Associate Professor of Clinical Medicine		
Arthur M. Feldman, MD	Clinical Associate of Medicine	PPMC	
Patricia A. Ford, MD	Director, Peripheral Stem Cell Transplant Program (PAH)	PAH	
	Director, Center for Bloodless Medicine and Surgery, PAH		
	Clinical Professor of Medicine		
Kevin R. Fox, MD	Mariann T. and Robert J. MacDonald Professor in Breast Cancer Care Excellence*	HUP	Breast

Name	Title	Location	Specialty (if applicable)
Noelle Frey, MD	Director of Clinical Cellular Therapy, Cell and Transplant Program	HUP	Leukemia/BMT
	Constance and Sankey Williams Associate Professor*		
Courtney Gabriel, MD	Clinical Associate in Medicine	CH	
Alfred L. Garfall, MD	Director, Autologous Hematopoietic Stem Cell Transplantation	HUP	Myeloma
	Assistant Professor of Medicine at the Hospital of the University of Pennsylvania		
James Gerson, MD	Assistant Professor of Clinical Medicine	HUP	Lymphoma
Saar I. Gill, MD, PhD	Assistant Professor of Medicine at the Hospital of the University of Pennsylvania	HUP	Leukemia/BMT/ Fundamental Research
Priva Gor, MD	Clinical Associate in Medicine	CH	
Richard Greenberg, MD	Section Chief, Hematology/ Oncology, Cherry Hill and Southern NJ	CH	
	Clinical Associate in Medicine		
Douglas E. Guggenheim, MD	Clinical Associate in Medicine	CH	
Naomi B. Haas, MD	Director, Prostate and Kidney Cancer Program	HUP	GU
	Professor of Medicine at the Hospital of the University of Pennsylvania		
Beatrice H. Hahn, MD	Professor of Microbiology	HUP	HIV/ Fundamental Research
	Professor of Medicine		

(Continued)

Name	Title	Location	Specialty (if applicable)
Gamil Hanna, MD	Medical Director, Infusion Services, Penn Medicine Cherry Hill Clinical Assistant Professor of Medicine	CH	GU
Lee Hartner, MD	Director, GI-CREP Program (PAH) Clinical Director, Sarcoma Medical Oncology (PAH) Clinical Associate Professor of Medicine	PAH	Sarcoma
Jessica Ann Hellyer, MD	Instructor A of Medicine	HUP	
David Henry, MD	Vice Chair, Department of Medicine (PAH) Clinical Professor of Medicine	PAH	HIV Malignancies
Maureen R. Hewitt, MD	Section Co-Chief, Hematology/Oncology, Chester County Hospital Clinical Associate of Medicine	CCH	
Elizabeth Hexner, MD	Medical Director, Center for Cellular Immunotherapies Associate Professor of Medicine at the Hospital of the University of Pennsylvania	HUP	Leukemia/BMT
Rebecca L. Hirsh, MD	Associate Professor of Clinical Medicine	HUP	
James A. Hoxie, MD	Professor of Medicine	HUP	HIV/Fundamental Research
Alexander Chanchi Huang, MD	Assistant Professor of Medicine	HUP	Melanoma

Name	Title	Location	Specialty (if applicable)
Rachel C. Jankowitz, MD	Director, Rena Rowan Breast Center	HUP	Breast
	Associate Professor of Clinical Medicine		
Yong Ji, MD	Clinical Associate of Medicine	CH	
Cheryl A. Johnson, MD	Clinical Associate of Medicine	CCH	
Thomas Karasic, MD	Assistant Professor of Medicine at the Hospital of the University of Pennsylvania	HUP	GI
Peter S. Klein, MD, PhD	Director, Physician Scientist Program	HUP	Benign Hematology/ Fundamental Research
	Professor of Medicine		
	Professor of Cell and Developmental Biology		
Hayley M. Knollman, MD	Assistant Professor of Clinical Medicine	HUP	Breast
Ingrid Kohut, DO	Clinical Assistant Professor of Medicine	PAH	
John A. Kosteva, MD	Clinical Assistant Professor of Medicine	VF	
Pallavi Kumar, MD, MPH	Director, Oncology Palliative Care	HUP	Palliative Care/GI
	Assistant Professor of Clinical Medicine		
Daniel J. Landsburg, MD	Vice Chief for Quality and Safety, Hematology/ Oncology	HUP	Lymphoma
	Assistant Professor of Clinical Medicine		
Corey J. Langer, MD	Director, Thoracic Oncology	HUP	Thoracic
	Professor of Medicine at the Hospital of the University of Pennsylvania		

(*Continued*)

Name	Title	Location	Specialty (if applicable)
Gerald P. Linette, MD, PhD	Clinical Director of the Parker Institute for Cancer Immunotherapy	HUP	Melanoma
	Chief Medical Officer for Cancer Immunotherapy		
	Professor of Medicine at the Hospital of the University of Pennsylvania		
Alison Wakoff Loren, MD, MS	Vice Chair, Faculty Development, Department of Medicine	HUP	Leukemia/BMT
	Director, Blood and Marrow Transplantation		
	Professor of Medicine at the Hospital of the University of Pennsylvania		
Selina M. Luger, MD	Professor of Medicine at the Hospital of the University of Pennsylvania	HUP	Leukemia/BMT
William E. Luginbuhl, MD	Section Co-Chief, Hematology/Oncology, Chester County Hospital	CCH	
	Clinical Associate of Medicine		
Carlos Madamba, MD	Clinical Associate of Medicine	CH	
Ivan P. Maillard, MD, PhD	Vice Chief for Research, Hematology/Oncology	HUP	Hematologic Malignancies/ Fundamental Research
	Professor of Medicine		
Robert G. Maki, MD, PhD	Clinical Director, Sarcoma Program	HUP	Sarcoma
	Professor of Medicine at the Hospital of the University of Pennsylvania		

Name	Title	Location	Specialty (if applicable)
Ronac Mamtani, MD, MSCE	Assistant Professor of Medicine at the Hospital of the University of Pennsylvania	HUP	GU
Melina Elpi Marmarelis, MD	Assistant Professor of Medicine at the Hospital of the University of Pennsylvania	HUP	Thoracic
Yehoda Martei, MD, MSCE	Vice Chief, Diversity, Inclusion and Health Equity, Hematology/ Oncology	HUP	Global Oncology
	Assistant Professor of Medicine at the Hospital of the University of Pennsylvania		
Lainie P. Martin, MD	Leader, Gynecology/ Oncology Program	HUP	Gynecologic
	Associate Professor of Medicine at the Hospital of the University of Pennsylvania		
Mary Ellen Martin, MD, FACP	Clinical Associate of Medicine	HUP	Leukemia/BMT
Ryan C. Massa, MD	Clinical Assistant Professor of Medicine	PPMC	GI
Kara N. Maxwell, MD, PhD	Assistant Professor of Medicine	HUP	Breast/Cancer Genetics/Fundamental Research
	Assistant Professor of Genetics		
Shannon R. McCurdy, MD	Assistant Professor of Medicine at the Hospital of the University of Pennsylvania	HUP	Leukemia/BMT
Kathryn A. McGrath, MD	Assistant Professor of Clinical Medicine	HUP	Palliative Care
David M. Mintzer, MD	Director, Palliative Care (PAH)	PAH	

(Continued)

Name	Title	Location	Specialty (if applicable)
	Section Chief, Hematology/ Oncology, PAH		
	Clinical Professor of Medicine		
Tara C. Mitchell (Gangadhar), MD	Associate Professor of Medicine at the Hospital of the University of Pennsylvania	HUP	Melanoma
Vivek K. Narayan, MD, MS	Assistant Professor of Medicine at the Hospital of the University of Pennsylvania	HUP	GU
Sunita Nasta, MD	Chair, Clinical Trials Review Monitoring Committee	HUP	Lymphoma
	Committee Chair, Penn Institutional Review Board		
	Associate Professor of Clinical Medicine		
Peter J. O'Dwyer, MD	Director, Developmental Therapeutics Program, Abramson Cancer Center	HUP	GI
	Professor of Medicine at the Hospital of the University of Pennsylvania		
Mark H. O'Hara, MD	Assistant Professor of Medicine at the Hospital of the University of Pennsylvania	HUP	GI
Vikram Ravindra Paralkar, MD	Assistant Professor of Medicine	HUP	Hematologic Malignancies/ Fundamental Research
	Assistant Professor of Cell and Developmental Biology		
James M. Patterson, MD	Clinical Associate of Medicine	CCH	

Name	Title	Location	Specialty (if applicable)
Alexander Perl, MD	Associate Professor of Medicine at the Hospital of the University of Pennsylvania	HUP	Leukemia/BMT
Allyson Pishko, MD, MSCE	Assistant Professor of Medicine at the Hospital of the University of Pennsylvania	HUP	Benign Hematology
David L. Porter, MD	Director, Cell Therapy and Transplantation	HUP	Leukemia/BMT
	Jodi Fisher Horowitz Professor in Leukemia Care Excellence*		
Keith W. Pratz, MD	Director, Leukemia Program	HUP	Leukemia/BMT
	Associate Professor of Medicine at the Hospital of the University of Pennsylvania		
Kim A. Reiss Binder, MD	Assistant Program Director of the Hematology/ Oncology Fellowship Program	HUP	GI
	Assistant Professor of Medicine at the Hospital of the University of Pennsylvania		
Kyle William Robinson, MD	Assistant Professor of Clinical Medicine	VA	
Marco Ruella, MD	Scientific Director of the Lymphoma Program	HUP	Lymphoma/ Fundamental Research
	Assistant Professor of Pathology and Laboratory Medicine		
	Assistant Professor of Medicine		

(*Continued*)

Name	Title	Location	Specialty (if applicable)
James Eric Russell, MD	Associate Professor of Medicine in Pediatrics	HUP	Benign Hematology/ Fundamental Research
	Associate Professor of Medicine		
Sunil Saroha, MD	Clinical Associate of Medicine	CCH	
Farzana Sayani, MD	Director, Penn Comprehensive Sickle Cell Program	HUP	Benign Hematology
	Director, Penn Comprehensive Adult Thalassemia Program		
	Assistant Professor of Medicine at the Hospital of the University of Pennsylvania		
Charles J. Schneider, MD, FACP	Clinical Professor of Medicine	HUP	GI
Lynn M. Schuchter, MD	Chief, Division of Hematology/Oncology	HUP	Melanoma
	Director, Tara Miller Melanoma Center		
	C. Willard Robinson Professor of Hematology-Oncology*		
Stephen J. Schuster, MD	Director, Lymphoma Program	HUP	Lymphoma
	Director, Lymphoma Translational Research		
	Robert and Margarita Louis-Dreyfus Professor in Chronic Lymphocytic Leukemia and Lymphoma Clinical Care and Research*		
Payal D. Shah, MD	Assistant Professor of Medicine at the Hospital of the University of Pennsylvania	HUP	Breast/Cancer Genetics

Name	Title	Location	Specialty (if applicable)
George M. Shaw, MD, PhD	Professor of Microbiology	HUP	HIV/Fundamental Research
	Professor of Medicine		
Lawrence N. Shulman, MD	Deputy Director, Clinical Services, Abramson Cancer Center	HUP	Breast
	Director, Center for Global Cancer Medicine, Abramson Cancer Center		
	Professor of Medicine at the Hospital of the University of Pennsylvania		
Aditi P. Singh, MD	Assistant Professor of Clinical Medicine	HUP	Thoracic
Edward A. Stadtmauer, MD	Section Chief, Hematologic Malignancies	HUP	Myeloma
	Roseman, Tarte, Harrow, and Shaffer Families' President's Distinguished Professor*		
Jakub Svoboda, MD	Associate Professor of Medicine at the Hospital of the University of Pennsylvania	HUP	Lymphoma
Samuel U. Takvorian, MD, MS	Assistant Professor of Medicine at the Hospital of the University of Pennsylvania	HUP	GU
Michele T. Tedeschi, MD	Clinical Associate of Medicine	CCH	
Ursina R. Teitelbaum, MD	Clinical Director, Penn Pancreatic Cancer Research Center	HUP	GI
	Deenie Greitzer and Daniel G. Haller Associate Professor*		
Donald Tsai, MD, PhD	Associate Professor of Medicine at the Hospital of the University of Pennsylvania	HUP	Lymphoma

(Continued)

Name	Title	Location	Specialty (if applicable)
David J. Vaughn, MD	Vice Chief for Clinical Affairs, Hematology/ Oncology	HUP	GU
	GU Medical Oncology Professor*		
Maria Vershvovsky, MD	Clinical Associate of Medicine	CCH	
Dan Vogl, MD	Director, Abramson Cancer Center Clinical Research Unit (CRU)	HUP	Myeloma
	Associate Professor of Medicine at the Hospital of the University of Pennsylvania		
Robert Herman Vonderheide, MD, DPhil	Director of the Abramson Cancer Center	HUP	Immunology/ Fundamental Research
	John H. Glick Abramson Cancer Center Professor*		
Kristine Marie Ward, MD	Clinical Assistant Professor of Medicine	PAH	
Max Miller Wattenberg, MD	Instructor A of Medicine	HUP	GI
Adam Waxman, MD, MS	Assistant Professor of Clinical Medicine	HUP	Myeloma
Yu-Ning Wong, MD	Associate Professor of Clinical Medicine	VA	GU
Stephen Zrada, MD	Clinical Associate of Medicine	CH	

Note: BMT = bone marrow transplant; CCH = Chester County Hospital; CH = Penn Cherry Hill; GI = gastrointestinal; GU = genitourinary; HIV = human immunodeficiency virus; HUP = Hospital of the University of Pennsylvania; PAH = Pennsylvania Hospital; PPMC = Penn Presbyterian Medical Center; VA = Veterans Affairs Hospital; VF = Valley Forge.

* Endowed professorships are noted with an asterisk.

Graduating Fellows of the Division of Hematology/Oncology (as of July 2021)

Year Completed	Name	Current Status
1974	Roger Anaya-Galindo	Academic, Universidad Juarez del Estado de Durango, Mexico
	Arnold Blaustein	Practice, Aventura, FL
	William Negendank	Deceased
1975	Rita Axelrod	Academic, Jefferson University
	Joel Bennett	Deceased
	DuPont Guerry IV	Academic, University of Pennsylvania, Retired
	Richard Rosenbluth	Practice, Teaneck, NJ
1976	Ross Abrams	Academic, Rush University
	Michael Karpf	Academic, University of Kentucky, Retired
1977	Alan Grosbach	Academic, University of Florida
	Martin Katz	Academic, Yale University
	James Kazura	Academic, University Hospitals Cleveland
	Nancy Scher	Food and Drug Administration

(*Continued*)

Year Completed	Name	Current Status
1978	Douglas B. Cines	Academic, University of Pennsylvania
1979	Gregory Favis	Practice, Daytona Beach, FL
	Paul Kaywin	Practice, Miami, FL
	Alvin Schmaier	Academic, University Hospitals Cleveland
1980	Janet Abrahm	Academic, Dana Farber Cancer Institute
	Anthony Bucolo	Practice, North Little Rock, AK
	Enrique Davila	Practice, Aventura, FL
	Arthur P. Staddon	Academic, University of Pennsylvania, Retired
1981	Roger Fleischman	Academic, University of Kentucky
	David Henry	Academic, University of Pennsylvania
1982	Mary Louise Kistner-Stone	Practice, Bluefield, WV
	Alan Lyss	Practice, St. Louis, MO
1983	Dennis Berman	Academic, University of Pennsylvania, Retired
	Francene Fleeger	Unknown
	Stanton Gerson	Academic, University Hospitals Cleveland
	Donna Glover	Deceased
	Peter Kovach	Practice, Springfield, OR
1984	Allan Davis	Practice, Lancaster, PA
	Lewis Rose	Academic, Jefferson University
1985	Joseph Kiss	Academic, University of Pittsburgh
1986	Steven C. Cohen	Practice, Bryn Mawr, PA, Retired
	Lawrence Flaherty	Academic, Wayne State University
	Alan Lichtin	Academic, Cleveland Clinic
	Susan Tannenbaum	Academic, University of Connecticut
1987	Brian Bolwell	Academic, Cleveland Clinic
	Daniel Brookoff	Deceased
	Kevin Fox	Academic, University of Pennsylvania
1988	Michel Hoessly	Practice, Paoli, PA, Retired
1989	Stephen Grabelsky	Practice, Boca Raton, FL

Year Completed	Name	Current Status
	David Grossman	Academic, Cleveland Clinic Florida
	Keith McCrae	Academic, Cleveland Clinic
	Edward Stadtmauer	Academic, University of Pennsylvania
	Ann Zimrin	Academic, University of Maryland
1990	Susan Kohler	Practice, Medford, OR
	Michael Spiritos	Academic, Duke University Health System
1991	James Chang	Unknown
	Deborah Ehrenthal	Academic, University of Wisconsin
	Michael Kolodziej	Industry, ADVI
	Marnin Merrick	Practice, Minot, ND
	Regina Resta	Practice, Troy, NY
	J. Eric Russell	Academic, University of Pennsylvania
	James Shaw	Academic, Medstar Health
1992	David Biggs	Practice, Newark, DE
	Neal Meropol	Industry, Flatiron Health
	Beth Overmoyer	Academic, Dana Farber Cancer Institute
	Sharona Sachs	Practice, Denver, CO
	Ralph Vassallo	Industry, Vitilant
1993	Selina Luger	Academic, University of Pennsylvania
	William Luginbuhl	Academic, University of Pennsylvania
	David Vaughn	Academic, University of Pennsylvania
1994	Robert DiPaola	Academic, University of Kentucky
	Rosemary Fiore	Practice, West Long Branch, NJ
	David Friedland	Academic, University of Pittsburgh
	Marc Kahn	Academic, University of Nevada, Las Vegas
	Michael Mikhail	Practice, Broomall, PA
	Robert Rotche	Practice, Blacksburg, VA
1995	Charles Schneider	Academic, University of Pennsylvania
	Newman Yielding	Industry, Janssen
1996	Victor Aviles	Practice, North Falmouth, MA

(Continued)

Year Completed	Name	Current Status
	Ken Laughinghouse	Practice, Little Silver, NJ
	Roberto Rodriguez	Practice, Pasadena, CA
	Warren Shlomchik	Academic, University of Pittsburgh
1997	Gowthami Arepally	Academic, Duke University
	M. Anne Blackwood-Chirchir	Industry, Innovators BioPharma Consulting, LLC
	Richard Greenberg	Academic, University of Pennsylvania
1998	Brenda Haynes	Practice, Wellesley, MA
	Alice Ma	Academic, University of North Carolina, Chapel Hill
	Gena Volas-Redd	Practice, Atlanta, GA
	John Wallmark	Practice, Rockville, MD
	Charles Whalen	Practice, Fort Wayne, Indiana
1999	Robert Green	Industry, Flatiron Health
	Edward Gunther	Academic, Pennsylvania State University
	Diane Hershock	Academic, Pennsylvania State University
	Clarissa Mathias	Academic, Brazil
	Halle Moore	Academic, Cleveland Clinic
2000	James Patterson	Academic, University of Pennsylvania
2001	Anna-Elina Armstrong	Academic, Helsinki, Finland
	Marcia Brose	Academic, Jefferson University
	Roy Kim	Practice, Madison, WI
	Ben Ho Park	Academic, Vanderbilt University
	Steven Stein	Industry, Incyte
	Weijing Sun	Academic, University of Kansas
	Nelson Yee	Academic, Pennsylvania State University
2002	Rebecca Elstrom	Industry, Fate Therapeutics Inc.
	Keith Flaherty	Academic, Massachusetts General Hospital
	Mary Ellen Martin	Academic, University of Pennsylvania
	Natalie Sacks	Industry, Harpoon Therapeutics
	Bradley Somer	Practice, Germantown, TN

Year Completed	Name	Current Status
2003	Tracy d'Entremont	Academic, University of Pennsylvania
	Julie Draznin Maltzman	Industry, Gilead Sciences
	Carl Henningson	Private Practice, Freehold, NJ
	James Thompson	Academic, Roswell Park
	Renee Ward	Industry, Loxo Oncology
2004	Charalambos Andreadis	Academic, University of California, San Francisco
	Ronald Buckanovich	Academic, University of Pittsburgh
	Hesamm Gharavi	Private Practice, Knoxville, TN
	Rebecca Kaltman	Academic, George Washington University
	Gregory Lubiniecki	Industry, Merck
	Ivan Maillard	Academic, University of Pennsylvania
	Kimryn Rathmell	Academic, Vanderbilt University
	Luisa Veronese	Industry, Roche
	Tal Zaks	Industry, Moderna Pharmaceuticals
2005	Joshua Bilenker	Industry, Treeline Biosciences
	Edwin Rock	Industry, Partner Therapeutics
	Kenneth Yu	Academic, Memorial Sloan Kettering Cancer Center
2006	Priya Gor	Academic, University of Pennsylvania
	Vandana Gupta Abramson	Academic, Vanderbilt University
	Molly Schachter Stumacher	Practice, Bryn Mawr, PA
2007	Anjali Avadhani	Academic, Jefferson University
	Maureen Hewitt	Academic, University of Pennsylvania
	Margaret Kasner	Academic, Jefferson University
	Magi Khalil	Practice, Gloucester, VA
	Roland Knoblauch	Industry, Janssen
	Ara Metjian	Academic, University of Colorado

(*Continued*)

Year Completed	Name	Current Status
2008	Sigrid Berg	Practice, Brewer, ME
	Mark Chiang	Academic, University of Michigan
	Anthony Mato	Academic, Memorial Sloan Kettering Cancer Center
	Benjamin Musher	Academic, Baylor College of Medicine
	Estelamari Rodriguez	Academic, University of Miami
	Marin Xavier	Academic, Scripps MD Anderson Cancer Center
2009	Arnob Banerjee	Industry, Janssen
	Jeremy Cetnar	Academic, Oregon Health and Science University
	Rachel Cook	Academic, Oregon Health and Science University
	Adam Cuker	Academic, University of Pennsylvania
	Esme Finlay	Academic, University of New Mexico
	Stephen Keefe	Industry, Merck
	Rebecca Olin	Academic, University of California, San Francisco
	Sophie Stein (Morse)	Practice, Summit, NJ
2010	Tapan Maniar	Industry, Dragonfly Therapeutics
	Rodolfo Perini	Industry, Merck
	Ran Reshef	Academic, Columbia University
	Matthew Riese	Deceased
	Jens Rueter	Academic, Jackson Laboratory
	Jared Weiss	Academic, University of North Carolina, Chapel Hill
	Jenia Jenab-Wolcott	Academic, Cooper University
2011	Brian Elliott	Practice, Mt. Kisco, NY
	Chunkit Fung	Academic, University of Rochester
	Keerthi Gogineni	Academic, Emory Winship Cancer Institute
	Karen Hook	Academic, University of Connecticut
	Jing-mei Hsu	Academic, Weill Cornell Medicine

Year Completed	Name	Current Status
	James Mangan	Academic, University of California, San Diego
	Sang Min	Academic, University of Michigan
	Emma Scott	Academic, Oregon Health and Science University
	Jennifer Shin	Academic, Massachusetts General Hospital
2012	Shannon Carty	Academic, University of Michigan
	Amy Clark	Academic, University of Pennsylvania
	Courtney DiNardo	Academic, M. D. Anderson Cancer Center
	Saar Gill	Academic, University of Pennsylvania
	Ronac Mamtani	Academic, University of Pennsylvania
	Vikram Paralkar	Academic, University of Pennsylvania
	Reshma Rangwala	Industry, Aravive
	Davendra Sohal	Academic, Cleveland Clinic
2013	David Bajor	Academic, University Hospitals Cleveland
	Joshua Bauml	Industry, Janssen
	Nicklas Pfanzelter	Academic, North Shore University Health
	Anjana Ranganathan	Practice, Bensalem, PA
	Alison Seghal	Academic, University of Pittsburgh
2014	Daria Babushok	Academic, University of Pennsylvania
	Christine Martin Ciunci	Academic, University of Pennsylvania
	Alfred Garfall	Academic, University of Pennsylvania
	Anita Kumar	Academic, Tufts Medical Center
	Daniel Landsburg	Academic, University of Pennsylvania
	Kara Maxwell	Academic, University of Pennsylvania
	Melissa Wilson	Academic, Jefferson University
2015	Orvar Gunnarsson	Academic, National University Hospital of Iceland
	Scott Huntington	Academic, Yale University
	Benjamin Jacobs	Practice, Media, PA
	Brandon Kremer	Industry, GlaxoSmithKline
	Marlise Luskin	Academic, Dana Farber Cancer Institute

(*Continued*)

Year Completed	Name	Current Status
	Jamin Morrison	Academic, Cooper University
	Mark O'Hara	Academic, University of Pennsylvania
	Nirav Shah	Academic, Medical College of Wisconsin
	Christian Squillante	Practice, Virginia Piper Cancer Institute
2016	Erin Aakhus	Academic, University of Pennsylvania
	Jonathan Canaani	Academic, Tel Aviv University, Israel
	Mark Diamond	Academic, University of Pennsylvania
	Alexander Huang	Academic, University of Pennsylvania
	Holleh Husseinzadeh	Academic, Jefferson University
	Vivek Narayan	Academic, University of Pennsylvania
	Robert Orlowski	Industry, Merck
	Mina Sedrak	Academic, City of Hope
2017	Stephen Bagley	Academic, University of Pennsylvania
	Thomas Karasic	Academic, University of Pennsylvania
	Yehoda Martei	Academic, University of Pennsylvania
	Sarah Nagle	Academic, Oregon Health and Sciences University
	Daniel Schreeder	Practice, Huntsville, AL
2018	Nina Beri	Academic, New York University
	Aaron Cohen	Industry, Flatiron Health
	Nathan Handley	Academic, Jefferson University
	Nicholas McAndrew	Academic, University of California, Los Angeles
	Christine McMahon	Academic, University of Colorado
	Allyson Pishko	Academic, University of Pennsylvania
	Pamela Sung	Academic, University of Pennsylvania
	Adam Waxman	Academic, University of Pennsylvania
2019	Adham Bear	Academic, University of Pennsylvania
	Elise Chong	Academic, University of Pennsylvania
	Tara Kaufmann	Academic, UT Health Austin
	Melina Marmarelis	Academic, University of Pennsylvania

Year Completed	Name	Current Status
	Ravi Parikh	Academic, University of Pennsylvania
	Joanna Rhodes	Academic, Northwell Health
	Nathan Singh	Academic, Washington University
	Sam Takvorian	Academic, University of Pennsylvania
2020	Emily Ayers	Academic, University of Virginia
	Steven Bair	Academic, University of Colorado
	Emily Feld	Academic, Memorial Sloan Kettering Cancer Center
	Christopher Manz	Academic, Dana Farber Cancer Institute
	Scott Peslak	Academic, University of Pennsylvania
	Max Wattenberg	Academic, University of Pennsylvania
	Jennifer Yui	Academic, Johns Hopkins University
2021	Zachary Frosch	Academic, University of Pennsylvania
	Amy Iarrobino Laughlin	Practice, Orlando, FL
	Kelsey Lau-Min	Academic, University of Pennsylvania
	Igor Makhlin	Academic, University of Pennsylvania
	Lova Sun	Academic, University of Pennsylvania
	Sandra Susanibar Adaniya	Academic, University of Pennsylvania
	Nathan Welty	Academic, University of Pennsylvania
	Shun Yu	Academic, University of Pennsylvania

NOTES

CHAPTER ONE

1. To Spread the Light of Knowledge: 250 Years of the Nation's First Medical School. Philadelphia: University of Pennsylvania Press, 2015.

2. Otto JC. An account of an hemorrhagic disposition in certain families. Med Reposit 1803;6:1.

3. Williams WJ, Esnouf MP. The fractionation of Russell's-viper (*Vipera russellii*) venom with special reference to the coagulant protein. J Biochem 1962;84:8452–62.

4. Nathan DG, Alter BP. Frank H. Gardner, MD (1919–2013). Hematologist 2013;10:4.

5. Schafer A, interview by D Vaughn (January 3, 2018). Interviews are cited on first mention in each chapter; subsequent quotations from the same person in the chapter are from the same source, unless otherwise noted.

6. Cooper III DY, Ledger MA. Innovation and Tradition at the University of Pennsylvania School of Medicine: An Anecdotal Journey. Philadelphia: University of Pennsylvania Press, 1990.

7. Kennedy BJ. Medical oncology: its origin, evolution, current status, and future. Cancer 1999;85:1–8.

8. Barker C, interview by D Vaughn (June 14, 2018).

9. Coggins PR, Ravdin RG, Eisman SH. Clinical evaluation of a new alkylating agent: cytoxan (cyclophosphamide). Cancer 1960;13:1254–1260.

10. Morning Call. "The Morning Call." October 9, 1963.

CHAPTER TWO

1. Glick J, interview by D Vaughn (November 8, 2017).

2. Cooper RA. Loss of membrane components in the pathogenesis of antibody-induced spherocytosis. J Clin Invest 1972;51:16–21.

3. Shattil S, interview by D Vaughn (November 15, 2017).

4. Abrams C, email communication (October 3, 2017).

5. Wiley JS, Ellory JC, Shuman MA, Shaller CC, Cooper RA. Characteristics of the membrane defect in the hereditary stomatocytosis syndrome. Blood 1975;46:337–356.

6. Wiley J, interview by D Vaughn (July 2018).

7. Alavi J, interview by D Vaughn (November 7, 2017).

8. Brass L, interview by D Vaughn (November 30, 2017).

9. Hoxie J, interview by D Vaughn (November 16, 2017).

10. https://ldi.upenn.edu/memoriam-pennldis-richard-buz-cooper (accessed June 30, 2021).

11. Cooper RL. Poverty and the Myths of Health Care Reform. Baltimore: Johns Hopkins University Press, 2016.

CHAPTER THREE

1. Glick J, interview by D Vaughn (November 8, 2017).

2. Alsop S. Stay of Execution: A Sort of Memoir. Philadelphia: JP Lippincott, 1973.

3. Bonnadonna G, Brusamolino E, Valagussa P, et al. Combination chemotherapy as an adjuvant treatment in operable breast cancer. N Engl J Med 1976;294:405–410.

4. Glick JH, Young ML, Harrington D. MOPP/ABV hybrid chemotherapy for advanced Hodgkin's disease significantly improves
failure-free and overall survival: the 8-year results of the intergroup
trial. J Clin Oncol 1998;16:19–26.

5. University of Pennsylvania Cancer Center Cancer Center Support
Grant (1974).

6. Abramson Cancer Center Cancer Center Support Grant (2020).

7. Nowell PC. Discovery of the Philadelphia chromosome: a personal
perspective. J Clin Invest 2007;117:2033–2035.

CHAPTER FOUR

1. Bennett J, interview by D Vaughn (November 14, 2017).

2. Lichtman MA, Spivak JL, Boxer LA, Henderson E, Shattil SJ.
Hematology: Landmark Papers of the Twentieth Century. London:
Academic Press, 2000.

3. Bennett JS, Vilaire G. Exposure of platelet fibrinogen receptors by
ADP and epinephrine. J Clin Invest 1979;64:1393–1401.

4. Bennett JS, Hoxie JA, Leitman SF, et al. Inhibition of fibrinogen
binding to stimulated human platelets by a monoclonal antibody.
Proc Natl Acad Sci USA 1983;80:2417–2421.

5. Hoxie J, interview by D Vaughn (November 16, 2017).

6. Popovic M, Sarngadheran MG, Read E, Gallo RC. Detection, isolation,
and continuous production of cytopathic retroviruses (HTLV-III) from
patients with AIDS and pre-AIDS. Science 1984;224:497–500.

7. Guerry D, interview by D Vaughn (November 21, 2017).

8. Guerry D, Kenna MA, Schrieber AD, Cooper RA. Concanavalin
A-mediated binding and sphering of human red blood cells by
homologous monocytes. J Exp Med 1976;144:1695–1700.

9. Mihm M, Clark WH. The clinical diagnosis, classification and
histogenic concepts of the early stages of cutaneous malignant
melanoma. N Engl J Med 1971;284:1078–1082.

10. Cines DB, Schreiber AD. Immune thrombocytopenia: use of a
Coombs antiglobulin test to detect IgG and C3 on platelets. N Engl J
Med 1979;300:106–111.

11. Cines DB, Kaywin P, Bina M, Tomaski A, Schreiber AD. Heparin-associated thrombocytopenia. N Engl J Med 1980;303:788–795.

12. Cuker A, Rux AH, Hinds JL, et al. Novel diagnostic assays for heparin-induced thrombocytopenia. Blood 2013;121:3723–3732.

13. Cuker A, Arepally G, Crowther MA, et al. The HIT Expert Probability (HEP) Score: a novel pre-test probability model for heparin-induced thrombocytopenia based on broad expert opinion. J Thromb Haemost 2010;8:2642–2650.

14. Brass L, interview by D Vaughn (November 30, 2017).

15. Glick J, interview by D Vaughn (November 8, 2017).

16. Haller D, interview by D Vaughn (December 6, 2017).

17. Moertel CG, Fleming TR, Macdonald JS, et al. Levamisole and fluorouracil for adjuvant therapy of resected colon carcinoma. N Engl J Med 1990;322:352–358.

18. Haller DG, Catalano PJ, Macdonald JS, et al. Phase III study of fluorouracil, leucovorin, and levamisole in high-risk stage II and III colon cancer: final report of Intergroup 0089. J Clin Oncol 2005;23:8671–8678.

19. Schmoll HJ, Tabernaro J, Maroun J, et al. Capecitabine plus oxaliplatin compared with fluorouracil/folinic acid as adjuvant therapy for stage III colon cancer: final results of the NO16968 randomized controlled phase III trial. J Clin Oncol 2011;33:1465–1471.

20. Alavi J, interview by D Vaughn (November 7, 2017).

21. Alavi JB, Root RK, Djerassi I, et al. A randomized clinical trial of granulocyte transfusions for infection in leukemia. N Engl J Med 1977;296:706–711.

22. Abrahm J, interview by D Vaughn (January 13, 2018).

23. Soros G. Reflections on death in America. Hosp J 1999;14:205–215.

CHAPTER FIVE

1. Shattil S, interview by D Vaughn (November 15, 2017).

2. Abrams C, interview by D Vaughn (November 9, 2017).

3. Luger SM, O'Brien SG, Ratajczak J, et al. Oligodeoxynucleotide-mediated inhibition of *c-myb* gene expression in autografted bone marrow: a pilot study. Blood 2002;99:1150–1158.

4. Abrams CS. Alan Gewirtz: a zest for life. Hematologist. January 31, 2011. https://ashpublications.org/thehematologist/article/doi/10.1182/hem.V8.1.1282/462241/Alan-Gewirtz-A-Zest-for-Life-1949-2010 (accessed September 24, 2018).

5. Glick J, interview by D Vaughn (November 8, 2017).

6. ASCO Daily News. "John H. Glick, MD, FASCO." 2009.

7. Glover D, Grabelsky S, Fox K, et al. Clinical trials of WR-2721 and cis-platinum. Int J Radiat Oncol Biol Phys 1989;16:1201–1204.

8. Fox K, interview by D Vaughn (December 7, 2017).

9. Consensus conference: adjuvant chemotherapy for breast cancer. JAMA 1985;254:3461–3463.

10. Stadtmauer E, interview by D Vaughn (November 28, 2017).

11. Stadtmauer E, O'Neill A, Goldstein LJ, et al. "Phase III Randomized Trial of High-Dose Chemotherapy (HDC) and Stem Cell Support (SCT) Shows No Difference in Overall Survival or Severe Toxicity Compared to Maintenance Chemotherapy with Cyclophosphamide, Methotrexate and 5-Fluorouracil (CMF) for Women." ASCO Annual Meeting. 1999.

12. Stadtmauer EA, O'Neill A, Goldstein LJ, et al. Conventional-dose chemotherapy compared with high-dose chemotherapy plus autologous hematopoietic stem-cell transplantation for metastatic breast cancer: Philadelphia Bone Marrow Transplant Group. N Engl J Med 2000; 342:1069–1076.

13. Stadtmauer EA, Fraietta JA, Davis MM, et al. CRISPR-engineered T cells in patients with refractory cancer. Science. 2020;367:eaba7365.

14. Schuchter L, interview by D Vaughn (August 28, 2018).

15. Schuchter L, Schultz DJ, Synnestvedt M, et al. A prognostic model for predicting 10-year survival in patients with primary melanoma: the Pigmented Lesion Group. Ann Intern Med 1996;125:369–375.

16. Halpern AC, Schuchter LM, Elder DE, et al. Effects of topical tretinoin on dysplastic nevi. J Clin Oncol 1994;12:1028–1035.

CHAPTER SIX

1. Mills OH Jr, Leyden JJ, Kligman AM. Tretinoin treatment of steroid acne. Arch Dermatol 1973;108:381–384.
2. Warrell RP Jr, Frankel SR, Miller WH Jr, et al. Differentiation therapy of acute promyelocytic leukemia with tretinoin (all-trans-retinoic acid). N Engl J Med 1991;324:1385–1393.

CHAPTER SEVEN

1. Shattil S, interview by D Vaughn (November 15, 2017).
2. Emerson S, interview by D Vaughn (December 5, 2017).
3. el-Deiry WS, Tokino T, Velculescu VE, et al. WAF1, a potential mediator of p53 tumor suppression. Cell 1993;75:817–825.
4. Wu GS, Burns TF, McDonald ER 3rd, et al. Induction of the TRAIL receptor KILLER/DR5 in p53-dependent apoptosis but not growth arrest. Oncogene 1999;18:6411–6418.
5. Porter DL, Roth MS, McGarigle C, Ferrara JL, Antin JH. Induction of graft-versus-host disease as immunotherapy for relapsed chronic myeloid leukemia. N Engl J Med 1994;330:100–106.
6. Porter D, interview by D Vaughn (March 1, 2018).
7. Couch FJ, Farid LM, DeShano ML, et al. *BRCA2* germline mutations in male breast cancer cases and breast cancer families. Nat Genet 1996;13:123–125.
8. Rebbeck TR, Friebel T, Lynch HT, et al. Bilateral prophylactic mastectomy reduces breast cancer risk in BRCA1 and BRCA 2 mutation carriers: the PROSE Study Group. J Clin Oncol 2004;22:1055–1062.
9. Rebbeck TR, Lynch HT, Neuhausen SL, et al. Prophylactic oophorectomy in carriers of BRCA1 or BRCA2 mutations. N Engl J Med 2002;346:1616–1622.
10. Klein P, interview by D Vaughn (July 2018).
11. Gurvich N, Tsygankova OM, Meinkoth JL, Klein PS. Histone deacetylase is a target of valproic acid-mediated cellular differentiation. Cancer Res 2004;64:1079–1086.

12. Carroll M, email communication with D Vaughn (June 28, 2021).

13. Schuster S, interview by D Vaughn (January 16, 2018).

14. Kastor JA. Governance of Teaching Hospitals. Baltimore: Johns Hopkins University Press, 2004

15. Staddon A, and Henry D, interview by D Vaughn (January 9, 2018).

CHAPTER EIGHT

1. Glick JH. "Overview of Abramson Cancer Center's Progress After the Transformational Gift from Madlyn and Leonard Abramson in Late 1997." 2018.

2. Kelley W, interview by D Vaughn (January 11, 2018).

3. Parmacek M, interview by D Vaughn (January 30, 2018).

CHAPTER NINE

1. Glick JH, email communication with D Vaughn (May 17, 2021).

2. Fox K, interview by D Vaughn (December 7, 2017).

3. DeMichele A, interview by D Vaughn (January 31, 2018).

4. Vonderheide R, interview by D Vaughn (December 12, 2017).

5. Domchek S, interview by D Vaughn (December 12, 2017).

6. Loren A, interview by D Vaughn (January 25, 2018).

7. Giantonio BJ, Catalano PJ, Meropol NJ, et al. Bevacizumab in combination with oxaliplatin, fluorouracil, and leucovorin (FOLFOX4) for previously treated metastatic colorectal cancer: results from the Eastern Cooperative Oncology Group Study E3200. J Clin Oncol 2007;25: 1539–1544.

8. Flaherty KT. Sorafenib in renal cell carcinoma. Clin Cancer Res 2007;13:747s–752s.

9. Flaherty KT, Lee SJ, Zhao F, et al. Phase III trial of carboplatin and paclitaxel with or without sorafenib in metastatic melanoma. J Clin Oncol 2013;31:373–379.

10. Davies H, Bignell GR, Cox C, et al. Mutations of the BRAF gene in human cancer. Nature 2002;417:949–954.

11. Flaherty KT, Puzanov I, Kim RB, et al. Inhibition of mutated, activated BRAF in metastatic melanoma. N Engl J Med 2010;363:809–819.

12. Chapman PB, Hauschild A, Robert C, et al. Improved survival with vemurafenib in melanoma with BRAF V600E mutation. N Engl J Med 2011;364:2507–2516.

13. Amaravadi R, Kimmelman AC, White E. Recent insights into the function of autophagy in cancer. Genes Dev 2016;30:1913–1930.

14. Karasic TB, O'Hara MH, Loaiza-Bonilla A, et al. Effect of gemcitabine and nab-paclitaxel with or without hydroxychloroquine on patients with advanced pancreatic cancer: a phase 2 randomized clinical trial. JAMA Oncol 2019;5:993–998.

15. University of Pennsylvania Almanac. "Director of the Abramson Cancer Center: Craig Thompson." September 19, 2006.

16. Emerson SP. "Department of Medicine Hematology Oncology Division Analysis and Review." 2006.

17. University of Pennsylvania Almanac. "President of Haverford College Stephen Emerson." February 20, 2007.

CHAPTER TEN

1. Shannon R, interview by D Vaughn (February 14, 2018).

2. Parmacek M, interview by D Vaughn (January 30, 2018).

3. Schuchter L, interview by D Vaughn (August 28, 2018).

4. Cohen R, interview by D Vaughn (January 8, 2018).

5. University of Pennsylvania Almanac. "Penn Medicine Advances Real-Time Medicine: The Ruth and Raymond Perelman Center for Advanced Medicine—Helping to Heal Patients Through Innovative Building Design." October 7, 2008.

6. Domchek S, interview by D Vaughn (December 12, 2017).

7. Domchek SM, Aghajanian C, Shapira-Frommer R, et al. Efficacy and safety of olaparib monotherapy in germline BRCA1/2 mutation carriers with advanced ovarian cancer and three or more lines of prior therapy. Gynecol Oncol 2016;140:199–203.

8. Kristeleit R, Shapiro G, Burris HA, et al. A phase I-II study of the oral PARP inhibitor rucaparib in patients with germline BRCA1/2-

mutated ovarian carcinoma or other solid tumors. Clin Cancer Res 2017;23:4095–4106.

9. ASH Clinical News. "Pulling Back the Curtain: Charles S. Abrams, MD." December 1, 2016. https://www.ashclinicalnews.org/features /pulling-back-the-curtain/charles-s-abrams-md (accessed September 25, 2018).

10. Cuker A, interview by D Vaughn (January 23, 2018).

11. George LA, Sullivan SK, Giermasz A, et al. Hemophilia B gene therapy with a high-specific-activity factor IX variant. N Engl J Med 2017;377:2215–2227.

12. Penn Medicine News. "Beatrice Hahn and George Shaw, Pioneers in HIV Research, to Join Penn Medicine." September 23, 2010. https://www.pennmedicine.org/news/news-releases/2010/september /beatrice-hahn-and-george-shaw (accessed September 27, 2018).

13. Tuma R. Two to the nth. Penn Medicine 2014;Winter:10–13.

14. Hahn BH, Shaw GM, Arya SK, Popovic M, Gallo RC, Wong-Staal F. Molecular cloning and characterization of the HTLV-III virus associated with AIDS. Nature 1984;312:166–169; and Shaw GM, Hahn BH, Arya SK, Groopman JE, Gallo RC, Wong-Staal F. Molecular characterization of human T-cell leukemia (lymphotropic) virus type III in the acquired immune deficiency syndrome. Science 1984;226:1165–1171.

15. Bernacki R, Hutchings M, Vick J, et al. Development of the Serious Illness Care Program: a randomised controlled trial of a palliative care communication intervention. BMJ Open 2015;5: e009032.

16. Staddon A, interview by D Vaughn (January 9, 2018).

17. Schuchter LM, email communication to Division (May 2018).

18. Berman D, interview by D Vaughn (February 14, 2018).

CHAPTER ELEVEN

1. Rosenberg SA, Packard BS, Aebersold PM, et al. Use of tumor-infiltrating lymphocytes and interleukin-2 in the immunotherapy of patients with metastatic melanoma: a preliminary report. N Engl J Med 1988;319:1676–1680.

2. Fox K, interview by D Vaughn (December 7, 2017).

3. Vonderheide RH, Dutcher JP, Anderson JE, et al. Phase I study of recombinant human CD40 ligand in cancer patients. J Clin Oncol 2001;19:3280–3287.

4. Beatty GL, Chiorean EG, Fishman MP, et al. CD40 agonists alter tumor stroma and show efficacy against pancreatic carcinoma in mice and humans. Science 2011;331:1612–1616.

5. Gangadhar TC, Hwu WJ, Postow MA, et al. Efficacy and safety of pembrolizumab in patients enrolled in KEYNOTE-030 in the United States: an expanded access program. J Immunother 2017;40:334–340.

6. Bagley SJ, Bauml JM, Langer CJ. PD-1/PD-L1 immune checkpoint blockade in non-small cell lung cancer. Clin Adv Hematol Oncol 2015;13:678–683.

7. Bellmunt J, de Wit R, Vaughn DJ, et al. Pembrolizumab as second-line therapy for advanced urothelial carcinoma. N Engl J Med 2017;376:1015–1026.

8. Parker Institute for Cancer Immunotherapy, website, https://www.parkerici.org/about/ (accessed September 28, 2018).

CHAPTER TWELVE

1. Thompson CB, Lindsten T, Ledbetter JA, et al. CD28 activation pathway regulates the production of multiple T-cell-derived lymphokines/cytokines. Proc Natl Acad Sci USA 1989;86:1333–1337.

2. Scholler J, Brady TL, Binder-Scholl G, et al. Decade-long safety and function of retroviral-modified chimeric antigen receptor T cells. Sci Transl Med 2012;4:132–153.

3. Porter DL, Levine BL, Kalos M, Bagg A, June CH. Chimeric antigen receptor-modified T cells in chronic lymphoid leukemia. N Engl J Med 2011;365:725–733.

4. Porter DL, Hwang WT, Frey NV, et al. Chimeric antigen receptor T cells persist and induce sustained remissions in relapsed refractory chronic lymphocytic leukemia. Sci Transl Med 2015;7:303ra139.

5. Loren A, interview by D Vaughn (January 25, 2018).

6. Maude SL, Frey N, Shaw PA, et al. Chimeric antigen receptor T cells for sustained remissions in leukemia. N Engl J Med 2014;371:1507–1517.

7. Frey NV, Porter DL. Cytokine release syndrome with novel therapeutics for acute lymphoblastic leukemia. Hematology Am Soc Hematol Educ Program 2016;2016:567–572.

8. Maude SL, Laetsch TW, Buechner J, et al. Tisagenlecleucel in children and young adults with B-cell lymphoblastic leukemia. N Engl J Med 2018;378:439–448.

9. Penn Medicine, https://www.facebook.com/pennmed/posts /10155017201187613 (accessed September 27, 2018).

10. Emily Whitehead Foundation, website, http:// emilywhiteheadfoundation.org/ (accessed September 28, 2018).

11. Emily Whitehead. "Carl June." Time.com, 100 Most Influential People 2018. http://time.com/collection/most-influential-people-2018 /5238121/carl-june/ (accessed September 28, 2018).

12. Schuster SJ, Svoboda J, Chong EA, et al. Chimeric antigen receptor T cells in refractory B-cell lymphomas. N Engl J Med. 2017;377:2545–2554.

13. University of Pennsylvania Almanac. "FDA Approves CAR T Therapy for Large B-Cell Lymphoma Developed at University of Pennsylvania." May 29, 2018.

EPILOGUE

1. Penn Medicine, Abramson Cancer Center, website. "Madlyn Abramson 1935–2020: The Passing of a Legend." https://www .pennmedicine.org/cancer/giving/about/madlyn-abramson-tribute (accessed June 30, 2021)

2. Jameson JL, Mahoney KB, email communication (May 19, 2021).

3. Abrams CS, email communication (June 21, 2021).

4. Abella BS, Jolkovsky EL, Biney BT, et al. Efficacy and safety of hydroxychloroquine vs placebo for pre-exposure SARS-CoV-2 prophylaxis among health care workers: a randomized clinical trial. JAMA Intern Med 2021;181:195–202.

5. Bange EM, Han NA, Wileyto P, et al. CD8+ T cells contribute to survival in patients with COVID-19 and hematologic cancer. Nat Med 2021;27:1280–1289.

6. Sun L, Sanjna S, Goodman NG, et al. SARS-CoV-2 seropositivity and seroconversion in patients undergoing active cancer-directed therapy. JCO Oncol Pract 2021;Jun 16:online ahead of print.

7. Singh AP, Berman AT, Marmarelis ME, et al. Management of lung cancer during the COVID-19 pandemic. JCO Oncol Pract 2020;16:579–586.

8. Cuker A, Tseng EK, Nierwlaat R, et al. American Society of Hematology 2021 guidelines on the use of anticoagulation for thromboprophylaxis in patients with COVID-19. Blood Adv 2021;5:872–888.

9. Zeidan AM, Boddu PC, Patnaik MM, et al. Special considerations in the management of adult patients with acute leukaemias and myeloid neoplasms in the COVID-19 era: recommendations from a panel of international experts. Lancet Haematol 2020;7:e601–612.

10. Ajai Chari A, Samur MK, Martinez-Lopez J, et al. Clinical features associated with COVID-19 outcome in multiple myeloma: first results from the International Myeloma Society data set. Blood 2020;136:3033–3040.

11. Bachanova V, Bishop MR, Dahi P, et al. Chimeric antigen receptor T cell therapy during the COVID-19 pandemic. Biol Blood Marrow Transplant 2020;26:1239–1246.

12. Penn Medicine, website. "The Pavilion." https://www.pennmedicine.org/for-patients-and-visitors/penn-medicine-locations/hospital-of-the-university-of-pennsylvania/pavilion (accessed June 30, 2021).

13. Schuchter L, email communication (June 16, 2021).

ACKNOWLEDGMENTS

I firmly believe that each of us makes one or two critical decisions that influence how our life evolves and who we become. The first and most important decision of my life was to marry Ann Leahey, my wife of thirty-five years. The second most important decision that I made was to come to the University of Pennsylvania to train in Hematology/Oncology and subsequently to join the faculty of the Division. It has been a privilege to work in the Division for over three decades, and I am grateful to my innovative and inspiring colleagues for all that you have done and all that you continue to do.

I especially want to express deep gratitude to Mattie Samuels-Crafton, my administrative assistant for over twenty years who recently retired. I am fortunate to work with three outstanding advanced practice providers: Barbara Zoltick, Linda Jacobs, and Caroline Pratz. Many thanks to my genitourinary oncology colleagues in the Division: Naomi Haas, Ronac Mamtani, Vivek

Narayan, and our latest recruit Sam Takvorian. I want to extend a special thank you to Vivek and Ron, who provided coverage for my three-month sabbatical when I wrote the first draft of this manuscript. I owe you both!

DuPont Guerry, Lynn Schuchter, and John Glick carefully reviewed this manuscript, and their suggestions have greatly enhanced its accuracy and readability. I am indebted to Mary Francis and her outstanding colleagues at Penn Press, who helped guide a novice through the publication process. Brian Ostrander and his colleagues at Westchester Publishing Services were instrumental in the production of this book. Many thanks to DeBalko Photography for granting me permission to include their photographs of the Division.

I want to thank my patients and their families, the main reason I come to work each day. Special thanks to Richard and Alison Prezelski, who with several other patients funded the Genitourinary Medical Oncology Professorship that I hold. Without this professorship, this project would not have been possible.

Many thanks to my parents, Bob and Barbara Vaughn of Rhode Island, who encouraged me to pursue my dream of becoming a physician.

To my wonderful twins, Erin and Luke, I could not love you more.

And, most importantly, I want to thank my astonishing wife, Annie. Your expertise in retinoblastoma, autism, and baseball are without equal.

Lightning Source UK Ltd.
Milton Keynes UK
UKHW012059240522
403466UK00004B/359